THE GOOD LIFE FOR CATS

health, happiness, and living on the edge

by Lee R. Harris, DVM

Dedicated to my patients, cat owners, my family, and my wife Terri.

ISBN 978-0-9861320-2-5 Print version
ISBN 978-0-9861320-3-2 eBook version

Keywords: 1. Cats-quality-of-life 2. Cats-health 3.Cats-behavior 4. Title

CONTENTS

Title Page

Dedications and copyright

Table of contents

Preface 1

  1. Life on the Edge 12

  2. Ways of Knowing 19

  3. Secret Senses 42

  4. Nothing More Than Felines 52

  5. A Sense of Place 64

  6. What's for Dinner 85

  7. Old and New Ways 103

  8. The Inside Story 115

  9. Let's Be Friends—Or Not! 135

10. Pandora's Problem 160

11. To the Good Life 175

12. Older and Wiser 205

Epilogue 228

Acknowledgements 232

References and reading 234

About the author 242

PREFACE

Ania, my black long-haired cat, sits perched on the back of the living room couch looking out the front window, her paws curled delicately under her chin and her eyelids half closed. It snowed last night, an uncommon occurrence in Seattle. The neighborhood sounds are muffled, giving the morning a deep sense of calm and peacefulness. As I watch Ania resting in her meditative pose, I wonder how she feels, what she thinks, and how she experiences the world on this snowy morning.

Trying to understand the inner life of a cat is more than an idle curiosity about a mind other than our own. It is difficult for me to imagine the thoughts of others, even people that I know and with whom I share common experiences, physiology, and culture. Understanding an animal's mind is speculative at best. But I have been a practicing veterinarian for forty years and my study of cats, neuroscience, and medicine has taught me that the relationship of cats with their world is critical to their health and happiness. When a client brings their kitty to my clinic with digestive problems, an infected bite wound, or a problem with urinating outside of the litter pan, many of my questions have to do with lifestyle: Food, household environment, activities, hidden stresses, social history, and the status of other cats in the house all hold vital clues to health and behavior.

This book is not about treating the diseases of cats; rather, we will explore how enriching the cat's experience and environment can improve its health. Because emotions and physical health are so intimately related, our journey will intersect with the common cat complaints at many points and the reader is asked to patiently tolerate excursions into the feline bladder, bowel, and hormones. The body has a lot to tell us. This is also not a book about treating behavior problems. Refusing to use the litter pan or sharpening claws on the good couch are distressing to the humans who share the cat's house, but these actions will concern us only because they are signposts to the cat's feelings. The mission of The Good Life For Cats is to examine the various elements of lifestyle and environment that influence feline health and happiness.

How can we understand how a cat feels about its world?

This book is an attempt to unravel these mysteries. I was prompted to begin this project after I published a book on canine lifestyle, "The Good Life for Dogs". But it quickly became apparent that investigating quality of life issues in cats would be much more difficult. Humans and dogs share similar social habits, dietary requirements, exercise needs, and communication channels, making it easy to understand our canine companions. Not so in cats. History has shown how the "otherness" of cats has been a source of human fascination, resulting in deification, vilification, and a million internet cat videos. Cats carry within them a certain wildness, even as we welcome them into our homes. We need to acknowledge that we can't always understand cats simply through intuition and empathy.

Since our own human experience is poorly equipped to comprehend the inner life of the cat, other tools are needed. Fortunately, science has provided a variety of different methods of investigation.

The science of animal behavior, termed ethology, studies how animals act. Data may be gathered from observations of wild beings in their natural habitat, close observation under captivity or domestication, and experimental studies. Each of these methods of discovery has its own shortcomings. In the wild, we only see a tiny fragment of an animal's life and context is impossible to establish. Nature documentaries show a lion bringing down a struggling wildebeest or fighting violently over territory. Nature, red in tooth and claw, but not really the stuff that dominates the daily life of a wild cat. Taking a long nap in the warm sunshine or gazing out over the plains may be more essential to the life of a wild lion than violent drama.

Keeping cats as pets allows us a much closer view of feline life, but much of the cat's mind is still hidden from us. Whether the cat feels anxious or serene, it keeps its feelings to itself.

In my patients I get a glimpse of the cat's mental experience when behavior problems occur. Nothing a cat does is ever accidental, whether it is urinating outside of the litter box or hissing at a familiar housemate "for no reason at all". Cats have their reasons, and a diligent search often reveals hidden motivations. If we really think we understand our cat's behavior, however, we may be led astray by anthropomorphism. Cats are complex conscious beings, but they are not human.

Animal psychologists have attempted to strip away the complexities of cat behavior by performing laboratory experiments that reduce the variables of everyday life. Unfortunately, these studies have often been misleading. One classic example involved an attempt to teach cats to press a lever for a food reward. A wide variety of animals from rats to chickens can learn this task easily, but when cats were tested they seemed unable to master this simple association. Scientists concluded that cats were just not smart enough. But when a cat was placed in a cage adjacent to another cat that would press the lever for food, the first cat immediately took to the task.[1] This result could be interpreted in a number of ways; the cat could lack the curiosity to try the lever, it could fail to make the connection between lever-pressing and food treats, it might be unable to learn a task by itself, or possibly it just might not be interested until someone else was doing it. The first three possibilities seem unlikely, given the inquisitive nature of cats and their uncanny ability to use any technique that gets results. Apparently the problem was not understanding, but motivation. The feline personality has often confounded behavior experiments in the lab.

Observation and experimentation have a lot to tell us, but we now have other ways of revealing what a cat may be thinking and feeling. The mind, whether human or feline, is governed by a host of hormones, neurotransmitters, and other molecules of emotion. These chemicals and their effects can be measured to show what the cat is feeling. Fear releases a surge of adrenaline, which raises the heart rate, blood pressure, and blood sugar levels, as well as alerting the body's "fight or flight" responses and prompting behavior change. Measure these reactions and we can guess what the cat is feeling. When the brain is forced to deal with change, a response we term "stress", cortisol is released into the bloodstream from the adrenal glands (prompted by the pituitary gland in the brain). We can inquire into what the cat is experiencing by measuring cortisol levels. The stress response is one of the most important influences on feline quality of life, so we will be discussing stress extensively in future chapters.

Peering even deeper into the brain with functional imaging (fMRI, PET scans) gives a spatial dimension to the mind. When we visualize the pathways that connect various parts of the brain, we can see emotion, motivation, and consciousness in action. Brain imaging helps to silence critics who claim that we are projecting our own feelings onto our cats. When we observe that our cat acts angry or fearful and similar areas of the feline brain light up on a fMRI as they do in a human under similar circumstances, it is difficult to claim that something fundamentally different is occurring.

The purpose of this book is to examine how we can improve the quality of life for the cats that share our lives. More than any other domestic species, behavior, physical health, and mental well-being are so intimately connected in the cat that they are often undistinguishable.

One of the most urgent examples of the convergence of mental and physical health involves urine. Every day in the veterinary hospital we examine cats that offend their owners by peeing outside of the litter box, and we have to sort through all of the possible factors to explain this distressing behavior. Infections or bladder stones may cause physical urgency to urinate, or an unpleasant frightening episode near the litter box may prompt avoidance behavior. The intrusion of a strange cat into the yard may trigger territorial marking behavior, or the diet of an overweight cat might raise the blood sugar enough to cause a prickly, painful sensation in the paws that makes stepping into the litter box uncomfortable. A surprising number of elimination problems respond to "environmental enrichment", but it is hard to know whether these interventions work by reducing stress, by allowing more natural behaviors, or simply by making the cat feel better inside. Often the answer is "all of the above".

One of the great mysteries of cats is that they can be easily upset by even the slightest change in their daily routine, but they can also invent creative new behaviors. It is the very complexity of feline behavior that attracts many

cat owners to their pets. Dogs show lots of interesting behaviors, but they tend to be drawn from a stock repertoire
of actions that combine natural dog-pack traits with useful
functions for which humans have selected. My clients are
usually either self-proclaimed "dog people", or "not dog
people", and the latter rarely become the former. Not so
with cats, however. A common scenario involves a "not-a-
cat-person" (often male), who becomes involved with a
"cat person" (typically female). At first the man will insist
that he has no use for cats, but he tolerates his romantic
partner's cat for her sake. But after a few months, he experiences a dramatic conversion. Now he is the one who
brings the cat to the vet for every little sniffle, and tells stories of the fascinating things that "his" cat does. The creative complexity of cat behavior makes cat lovers out of
normal people. This raises the question of how a creature
that craves stability and routine is able to leap out of its
natural behaviors and adapt to life with people, cats, dogs,
and the chaotic human environment in which they willingly
find themselves.

Several comments are in order before we explore the
world of cats. The first has to do with terminology: Some
animal advocates will object to the use of the word "owner"
to refer to people who keep cats. It is frequently observed

that cats act like they own us, rather than the other way around. Our relationship with cats is a mutual contract, and referring to a "cat owner" is not meant to imply that cats are our slaves, servants, or inferior beings. In the veterinary hospital, we use the term "owner" to indicate who is paying the bill. Our relationship with cats may be equal and symbiotic, but for brevity and simplicity we will refer to cat owners. Don't read too much into the words.

In my book about lifestyle and dogs, I drew upon anecdotes and observations of my canine patients to illustrate the lifestyle principles under discussion. This turns out to be much more difficult in cats. These pages will include lots of stories and observations of real cats, but most of them are drawn from my personal cats and those of family members. I see my feline patients when their lives are at their worst, making it hard to discern what makes them happy and content. Dog owners can intuitively explain their pet's likes and dislikes, but cats are simply more opaque in their health and behavior. Understanding why cats feel and react the way they do requires close daily contact combined with all the medical knowledge we can muster. I have frequently been fooled by my own cats, and often the key that explains a health or behavior change occurs only as a fleeting glimpse: A different sleeping spot or restless behavior at night may be the only clue we have. Observing more than two dozen of my own cats and those of close friends has provided helpful hints to understanding the thousands of other cats that I have had the privilege to treat in my hospital. My own cats will be given their real names, while my clients' pets will have their names changed. But these observations only scratch the surface of feline behavior. Every reader will know that their own cat does things that are not explained in these pages; not every mystery can be explained.

Finally, this book is necessarily written in the first person. Although I will draw on the feline scientific literature (which is much more sparse than the research on dogs) and the writings of naturalists, animal rescue workers, and devoted cat people, these sources are filtered through my own experience of treating over fifty thousand cat patients in health and disease. This personal experience with cats is central to my understanding of how we can make life better for cats. I will attempt to separate my opinions and speculation from the scientific facts gathered by other veterinarians and researchers.

Exploring the inner lives of cats should open our minds to the possibilities of other ways of perceiving the world. Anthropologists do this when attempting to understand other cultures, psychiatrists do this when they probe the experiences of bipolar or autistic patients, and teachers do this when they try to connect with students who are blind, deaf, or cognitively impaired. By exploring the inner lives of cats, we may be able to improve the quality of life for our pets. We may even learn a little about our lives along the way.

Chapter 1: LIFE ON THE EDGE

In the tall grass of a small clearing in Tanzania, an imperceptible movement suddenly erupts into a series of three leaps as a tawny wildcat pounces on a small antelope, which she subdues after an intense struggle. The wildcat is a caracal, thirty pounds of sleek feline muscle and motion, but she has to overcome a disadvantage of twenty pounds and two sharp horns as she fights for her dinner. The struggle over, she barely catches her breath before carrying her prize to her den. She noticed that the grass just up the track had been flattened by a larger animal, possibly a hyena lurking nearby to rob her of her kill, so she hurries with her catch to the shelter of a nearby hill. The hot African sun is just starting to warm up the savanna as she drops her prey in front of the four kittens that she had hidden in a rocky outcropping. As the mother cat watches her kittens attack the meal that she brought them she glances around frequently, her tufted ears erect and alert; the previous evening she had heard sounds of two wildcats fighting, and she knew that any strange male who moved into the area was a danger to her kittens. Should she move her family to a new location, or try to stay inconspicuous and observe the surrounding territory for a day or two and assess the situation? These decisions mean the difference between life and death, with little room for mistakes. And yet, the graceful wildcat appears to be calm and relaxed as she sprawls over her lookout spot, watching with lidded eyes. No wasted motion here, no nervous pacing, no outward sign that all of her internal systems are poised to spring into action if anything changes.

Biologists have a name for the body's response to change: Stress. When action needs to be taken to deal with a sudden change, the nervous system immediately lights up in a flurry of activity as it analyzes the situation and readies the body for action. Blood pressure and heart rate increase, in case the muscles are called upon to make a speedy escape or an aggressive rush. Pupils dilate to collect and interpret any relevant visual information. Blood sugar increases to turbocharge the brain and the muscles.

In her wonderful book, "The Tribe Of Tiger"[A], Elizabeth Marshall Thomas describes how the entire cat family evolved for "life on the edge". The ancestors of our house cats adopted a life that allowed no compromise. All cats are obligate carnivores that can only subsist on what they catch, requiring incredible senses and physical abilities in order to survive. While other predators like wolves, bears, and humans can forage for edible plants during lean times and are able to synthesize many necessary nutrients from other available sources, cats have unusually demanding dietary requirements. Feline species have adapted to some of the most unforgiving environments on earth, from the snows of Siberia and the Himalayas to the deserts of Africa, Asia, and the American Southwest. Water is often sparse or absent, so the cat's body must be able to create and conserve every drop of water in order to survive. Resources are precious and the cat must use any means possible to protect its territory. If marking with urine, feces, and claw marks are not enough, the wild cat must be willing to use its teeth, claws, and voice to defend its homeland. The cat family has risen to these challenges with sharp intelligence, physical prowess, and acute senses, but these all come at a cost.

Cats are the ultimate stress-driven creature, adapted to life on the edge, and it is impossible to discuss the feline experience without understanding how stress affects the body and mind. Stress and change have both positive and negative effects on the quality of the cat's life with humans, a theme to which we will return frequently throughout this book as we seek to understand our feline companions.

Stress isn't necessarily distressing. We might even conclude that thriving in response to change is the essence of life. Cats are destined by nature to handle challenges that would be impossible for an animal of less intelligence or limited physical prowess, and cats seem to enjoy using these abilities. Short-term stress responses can feel good, make us feel more alive, and allow our neuroendocrine systems to do what they were meant to do.

While a little stress can be a good thing, the capacity to deal with change has its limits. Veterinarians frequently observe the consequences of a cat's inability to deal with changes, great and small. The most obvious sign of stress is the nervousness that most cats experience when a bumpy car ride in a small plastic carrier ends in a noisy waiting area, where the sounds and smells of strange people, dogs, and cats mingle with the odors of disinfectants and medications. By the time the veterinarian extracts the kitty from its carrier, everyone in the room is tense. The cat's short-term stress response can make it hard to get accurate vital signs: The heart rate, which was 120 beats per minute at home, is closer to 200. Blood pressure is difficult enough to measure on tiny little cat legs, but in the veterinary hospital we know that it will soar above normal. Cats' stress responses are so robust that blood sugar may elevate above 250 when nervous, a level that would be considered diabetic in a person or a calm cat. In the past veterinarians tended not to handle cats gently and respectfully, but during the last decade advocates in our profession have reminded us that cats have a hard enough time as it is, and they deserve as little stress as possible when medical care is needed. No matter how kind and gentle the veterinary staff is, any visit to the hospital is stressful. Fortunately, the cat's emergency responses recover quickly from stress that only lasts an hour or two.

When stress continues for days and weeks, especially when the cat has no ability to control the sources of challenge and change, natural coping abilities are strained and mental and physical health are affected. Veterinarians are starting to understand how stress can affect cats: Young cats with inflammation of the bladder, middle aged cats with inflammation of the intestine, and bald cats with a compulsive over-grooming condition termed "psychogenic alopecia" all suffer from problems that have been associated with changes in the cat's environment. Questions about the patient's lifestyle have become part of almost every feline office call.

"But my cat has nothing to be stressed about!", cat owners respond when queried about changes in the cat's routine. "All he does is sleep all day and demand his favorite food on his own schedule, which I always give him". The person may indeed be providing food, water, and affection, but be blissfully unaware of the concerns of a sensitive animal trying to live in an overstimulating human environment with minimal control over its situation. Even rearranging the living room furniture impacts the cat's nervous system as it tries to understand why the couch is in a different corner and how it should handle this new configuration. Indoor cats are very attuned to activity in the neighborhood, and many times I learn that the inside cat who appears to have an idyllic life starts urine marking just after a stray tomcat has been seen in the area. We will see in future chapters how sounds, smells, and vibrations that are imperceptible to humans can affect the well-being of our cats.

One thing that is obvious is that cats vary a lot in how they handle stress. For some cats, excitement and change are a tonic, while in other cats they cause debilitating physical and psychological problems. The difference in theses cats can be traced to the beginnings of kittenhood. Hundreds of studies[1,2,3,4,5] have shown that the balance of stress hormones and the neurotransmitters that respond to change can be altered permanently by the attention that the mother lavishes on her young, or even by the stress that she experiences before her babies are born. This is a significant factor when we adopt a kitten that was an orphan, rescued from a feral mother, or spent its early weeks in a shelter environment. We may not know what early life was like for a kitten that we adopt, but these early experiences are etched into the cat's nervous system, creating resilience or vulnerability to future stress.

During future chapters we will examine many of the factors that affect the daily lives of cats, ways to reduce stress, and when stress is good for your cat. But first, we need to imagine how the cat's exquisite senses influence how life is experienced in the feline mind.

Chapter 2: WAYS OF KNOWING

"Where is Oscar this morning?", asks a woman in teal-colored scrubs. Her inquiry is the most frequent question asked during shift change at this Rhode Island nursing home. Oscar lives at the facility for advanced dementia patients, along with several other pets. The gray and white shorthaired cat had been adopted as a kitten to serve as a companion and therapy cat for the patients, but he turned out to be a generally unsociable addition to the nursing home staff. Except when a person was near death, that is. When Oscar hops up on one of the beds to curl up with a frail elderly patient, the staff knows that the end of life is near. At first the doctors and nurses were skeptical that a cat could sense the approach of death more accurately than the medical staff, but after more than fifty documented episodes it became clear that this unexceptional kitty knew when death was coming, and he was compelled to spend these last hours purring and snuggling with the soon-to-be-deceased.

Oscar's story was first recounted in the New England Journal of Medicine in 2009 by Dr. David Dosa, a gerontologist who works at the nursing home. As more patients were added to the list, Dr. Dosa described his observations in a moving book, "Making Rounds With Oscar: The Extraordinary Gift Of An Ordinary Cat"[B]. There is no doubt that this cat had a "sixth sense" (or maybe that should be a ninth or tenth sense) for the ebbing of life, but Dr. Dosa was unable to explain how Oscar knew. Other cats that had lived in the facility never showed the same behavior, but perhaps they simply noted the patient's condition and kept it to themselves.

The word "mysterious" inevitably appears in any description of the sensing abilities of cats. Often a lack of scientific explanation leads to other descriptions: "supernatural", "paranormal", "ESP", and even "occult". The inability to explain cat behavior has fascinated humans for millennia, and often not in a good way.

The mysterious perceptual abilities of cats made them gods in ancient Egypt, but their reputation went downhill from there. By the Middle Ages the secret ways of feline knowledge were more feared than admired. Cats were thought to be spies and advisors to witches, perhaps even witches themselves, leading to the persecution and slaughter of thousands of unfortunate animals. Black cats were particularly reviled, and even now black cats are much less likely to be adopted from shelters than cats of other colors[1]. Ironically, some studies of coat color and personality have shown that black cats are often more docile and more willing to hang out with humans than cats of other hues. It isn't fair, but people often tend to react badly to things that we don't understand.

If we accept that cats are endowed with their own form of consciousness, we have to ponder the question of what their experience is like. Philosopher Thomas Nagel addressed this problem in a famous 1974 essay entitled "What Is It Like To Be A Bat?"[2]. Nagel wasn't really concerned with the daily life of flying mammals, but rather with "the subjective character of experience" for each sentient being. His philosophical argument insisted that every conscious being has their own unique and private sphere of experience, and no matter how much we comprehend of the mental processes behind the mind, we can't really know how it feels to be another person or animal. This suggests that the cat's world is hidden to us, even if we try to imagine that we could see in the dark or hear the ultrasonic chirps of mice. And yet, the question of what life is like for a cat (and how we can make it better) is the central theme of this book. Let's think about this.

One of Nagel's points is that reducing life to its component parts fails to capture the whole that makes up subjective experience. With the reader's indulgence, I will take the liberty of pondering how the cat's incredibly acute senses combine to create feline awareness, before moving on to explore what we know about the individual senses. Then we can consider the practical implications of how the environment that we provide affects our cat's quality of life.

My interest was aroused when I learned that the nerve signals from the cat's touch-sensitive whiskers accompany the nerve signals from the eyes on their way to the areas of the brain where "seeing" occurs. The whiskers, or vibrissae, are remarkable organs in their own right. These long stiff hairs frame the cat's face, as well as protruding above the eyes and near the elbows. Whiskers are richly supplied with specialized touch receptors and serve a number of functions that we are able to identify. They offer protection around the eyes by sensing approaching objects in time for the cat to blink, a useful feature for an animal that is active in the dark. Since the whiskers on the face extend to an area approximately the size of the cat's body, we assume that they help the cat test the size of an opening to see whether the rest of the body will be able to pass through. But most impressive is that the vibrissae are extremely sensitive to faint air currents, complimenting the feline ability to "see" in the dark. The flow of air reflects the texture and position of surrounding surfaces as well as temperature of the immediate area, allowing the brain to create a spatial representation. If a cat with perfectly intact whiskers is placed in a completely dark room, it will move confidently and avoid obstructions easily. If the same cat has damaged vibrissae, it will proceed tentatively, unable to sense its surroundings.

Although cats are active at night, roaming and hunting, their world is rarely in complete darkness. Feline eyes are adapted to make the best use of the faintest glimmer of light, and although their color vision is not as complete as ours, the red-sensing cones in the retina respond to wavelengths beyond red, the same infra-red radiation that is used in high-tech heat-imaging cameras. When the motion-sensing ability of the whiskers is combined with ultra-sensitive vision, the result is a "night vision" that is actually a composite of several senses. Once smell and acute hearing are added to the cat's toolbox, it isn't surprising that cats seem to know more about their environment than we can comprehend. But what does this seem like to the cat?

It is tempting to think about each of our senses as separate entities, and when we test the senses we attempt to isolate each of them from the others. When the eye doctor asks us to read the bottom line on the eye chart, she doesn't expect us to sniff the chart or reach out and touch the letters. Studying the senses in isolation allows us to determine the limits of each individual sense, but it may not reflect how the mind experiences its environment.

The brain, human or feline, has specialized areas to process input from different sensors. The visual cortex for sight, auditory centers for hearing, etc. But these channels are not completely separate. To varying degrees, the five familiar senses are adapted to be used as a whole. What we hear is affected by what we see, and taste is actually a combination of taste, smell, and the texture and temperature reported by nerve endings in the mouth.

An extreme example of the combination of the senses is synesthesia, which occurs in as many as five percent of humans. To the synesthete, a sound may be accompanied by the perception of a specific color, or a bitter taste may create the physical sensation of touching a sharp object. Synesthesia is likely more common than we realize, since many people keep this merging of sensations to themselves, lest they be thought weird. To a person with synesthesia the senses act as a committee, rather than operating separately.

I am speculating here, but my personal intuition is that the cat's acute senses are less separate then we imagine, something closer to synesthesia. If we were able to ask the cat how it "sees" in the dark, it might say that it "just knows" where surrounding objects are. People who are blind can learn to hear faint high-pitched echoes from surrounding surfaces and feel the surface beneath their feet with an outstretched cane. Even though the sightless person is using hearing and touch to navigate, they often report that it is "something like seeing", with indistinct images that are experienced in a visual sort of way. More recently, neuroscience has confirmed this observation, showing that the areas of the brain specialized for vision, touch, and hearing are able to receive and interpret input from other senses as well. And there are other hints that cats might merge their senses in some manner.

Buried in the midbrain lies a structure called the superior colliculus. The specialized sensory areas of the brain send information about vision, hearing, touch, and other senses to the superior colliculus, where this information forms overlapping sensory maps. In this area, each of these inputs is modified by information from the other senses[3]. For instance, if visual input suggests that something is worthy of attention, it may amplify the input from the touch receptors for the relevant area. This combined information is then fed to multi-modal neurons and forwarded to the cortex for action. The combination of sensations in the superior colliculus creates a multiplying effect that far exceeds the ability of any single sense. It is hard to know whether a cat is consciously aware of individual sensory stimuli, or whether the combined senses create a "supersense" by combining their interacting inputs. My personal suspicion is that the "supernatural" ability of cats to know the world rests on a greater interaction of the senses. From this perspective we can conjecture how a cat like Oscar might sense the approach of the end of a human life, using combinations of the familiar five senses.

Seeing is believing, or so most humans believe. Are there visual cues that tipped Oscar to the loss of his patient's hold on life? Perhaps Oscar could see life slipping away by noticing subtle visible changes in the skin and eyes. Doctors may be trained to measure blood pressure and check an EKG, but the subtleties of "You don't look so good" may be lost on a highly trained physician. The color of the skin reflects the capillary circulation on the body's surface, which changes before a stethoscope can tell that the heart is beating its last. The feline ability to see light wavelengths in the infra-red range adds a temperature dimension, and the skin would start to cool slightly before the core body temperature drops. Vision also reveals the texture and elasticity of the skin, which change along with the body's hydration.

The cat's visual abilities are legendary. The eyes are proportionately large, with highly curved corneas to provide a wide field of vision. The light sensitive retina uses an efficient method to amplify the light that shines on the back of the eye: A shiny reflective surface called the tapetum lucidum produces the familiar green glow-in-the-dark appearance of the feline eye by reflecting incoming light after it passes through 15 layers of light-sensing neurons. Each photon stimulates the vision cells and then bounces back through the retina to stimulate the cells again. A neat trick, catching light coming and going,

Most mammals possess two types of light receptors in the retina: The rods, which are very sensitive and can operate in low light (but don't register color), and the cones, which require more light (but can distinguish the different wavelengths of light). Cats have a greater number of the sensitive rods, useful for an animal that is active at dusk and darkness. There are fewer color-responsive cones, and most of these are tuned to green wavelengths of light. There are also some cones that are triggered by blue, and some that sense beyond the red end of the human visual spectrum, in the infra-red zone radiated by body heat. Infra-red cameras are used in the military to identify the presence of people or other warm objects in total darkness, an ability that cats find useful in their nocturnal activity.

In addition to the tricks that the feline eye does with light, the visual cortex can perform complex calculations with the nerve signals arriving from the eyes. The brain selectively searches for sudden changes, indicating movement. In a stationary scene, much of the information is ignored; a still-life picture isn't very useful to a predator. But when a sudden change in visual motion is sensed, the brain (and even certain layers of the retina) starts comparing and analyzing to produce a high-definition image. The faintest twitch of a mouse's tail under a pile of leaves stands out in bold contrast.

Let's return to touch and the whiskers. The vibrissae are richly supplied with nerves that sense any movement of the whisker, whether it is brushing up against the edge of a rodent's burrow or feeling a stirring of air currents on a calm night. These impulses are relayed to the brain along the same paths as visual signals, although we don't know how much the two senses are mixed together as they travel. Whether signals from the whiskers form part of the picture in the visual cortex or they are added to the mix later in the superior colliculus, the combination of vision and touch give an image that is rich in information.

Touch is certainly not confined to the whiskers. The cat's entire body has nerve endings for several types of stimulation. Pain sensors (called nociceptive receptors) report a sharp reaction to injury and inflammation, heat-sensitive nerves monitor temperature, and pressure recep-tors sense when the skin is rubbed, tapped, or petted.

One of the most interesting aspects of the cat's skin is how they sense heat. As humans we find it uncomfortable when we touch an object that is over 112 degrees F. But the heat-sensing nerve endings of the cat don't start to complain until the temperature reaches 126 degrees F, which would be enough to make a person say "Ouch!" and withdraw. This difference is obvious when we observe our cat stretched out comfortably in front of the fireplace on a winter evening. Reaching out to pet the cat, we find that its fur is uncomfortably hot to our touch, although the cat ap-pears unconcerned. This makes sense in an animal that evolved in hot environments like the Sahara Desert; one can imagine a wildcat hunting for mice along a sand dune in Egypt on a sunny day and walking gingerly across the hot sand meowing "Ohh! Ahh! Ow!"—not a good way to catch dinner.

Heat-detecting receptors are particularly plentiful on the hairless surface at the tip of the cat's nose, an area called the planum nasale. These heat sensors may work along with the whiskers to provide a thermal picture of anything that might be right in front of the cat's nose. These nerves can detect temperature differences of less than .9 degrees F, which would allow Oscar to gauge a person's skin temperature as well as a thermometer.

The touch receptors in the loose skin over the cat's shoulders produce their own peculiar reaction. In very young kittens, pinching the scruff of the neck causes a sudden paralysis-like relaxation of the body. This reflex prevents the kittens from squirming around when a mother cat picks up her babies to move them to a new den. This response tends to disappear with age, although we will occasionally see a kitten go limp for a few seconds after an injection is given over the shoulder area. In one novel application of this phenomenon, a soft plastic "scruff clip" is used by some veterinarians to produce a temporary calming reaction during a minor procedure (like drawing a blood sample). The cats don't seem to mind, and there is good evidence that scruff clips can be effective in some cats. This same reasoning is sometimes used to falsely justify "scruffing" a cat by grabbing a handful of loose skin for restraint. Cats hate this, and they are slow to forgive anyone who treats them in this way.

The cat's body has fewer touch nerve endings than a person, reflecting the fact that our skin is exposed and needs to react to the slightest stimulus to protect ourselves. The cat's dense layer of fur muffles the sensation of touch, as well as the vulnerability to minor scrapes and scratches. The pads of the paws have lots of nerves, which may help the cat walk silently when it chooses. In Chapter 12 we will see how this can cause a cat to suffer when these nerves become hypersensitive due to high blood sugar.

The intimate relationship between the brain and the sense of touch is involved in a poorly understood condition termed the Feline Hyperesthesia Syndrome. Occasionally we will see cats that are so sensitive to touch that they will fall over and twitch when petted over the rump area. Even the contact of the cat's own tongue with the skin can trigger a seizure-like reaction and self-inflicted bites. In some cases it appears to be triggered by a skin problem such as flea bite allergy, but in other cases it seems more like a type of epilepsy in which a brainstorm is triggered by normal sensations. To make things even more confusing, the reactions of these cats overlap with some normal behaviors, such as sexual stimulation, kitten hyperactivity, or self-induced excitement ("seeing spacemen"). When brain waves are recorded during an episode they show tracings somewhere in between a seizure, normal activity, and a transition into the sleep state. What is clear is that the behavior is pathologic when it turns self-destructive. This syndrome reminds us that the sense of touch is not to be taken lightly; the feeling of contact can be heavenly or hellish.

One of the most plausible explanations for Oscar's uncanny ability to anticipate death lies in the cat's sense of smell. Humans are pitiful underachievers when it comes to sensing the environment through our noses, and most of our olfactory receptors lie in the back of the nasal cavity where they are best suited for sampling aromas from our food as we chew it. Cats have more smell receptors and they are strategically positioned forward in the convoluted nasal passages. Here odor molecules are concentrated and sorted to detect the scent of prey and the olfactory communications of other cats. Just as we cannot know what it is like to be a bat, we cannot know what it is to smell our environment in the same way that a cat does.

There is no doubt that there are many smells that tell of sickness, and of death. Even human doctors can sometimes get a whiff of some specific disease. The smell of acetone on the breath reveals the presence of ketones from uncontrolled diabetes, and the ammonia-like smell of urea waste products suggests kidney failure.

Dogs are more famous than cats for their ability to scent infections, cancer, and diabetes, but this could be because dogs are more willing to tell us what they are smelling. The feline nose may not be able to compete with a trained canine sniffer, but even the average cat can tell a lot about us by our scents. In addition to the chemical imbalances of disease, the smell of our breath, our skin, and our urine provides a detailed picture of health.

It is likely that cats can also smell many of our major hormones, from cortisol to testosterone and estrogen, to minor hormones like melatonin, adrenalin, insulin-like growth hormone, thyroxine, oxytocin, and dozens of other chemical messengers in our bodies. Sensing these hormones, singly or in combination, could have told Oscar which patient was poised on the brink of death. The scent of these hormones can also communicate our moods to our pets. More melatonin is produced when we are sleepy, and testosterone spikes when men watch their favorite team win a football game. It may seem like cats can read our minds, but they may be smelling our emotions. Even if the miniscule amounts of our circulating hormones cannot be detected by the cat, chemical changes in our skin secretions may reveal what our hormones are doing. When our body chemistry reacts to a stressful stimulus, the content of our sweat changes in ways that would be obvious to the cat's nose. Some of these same changes are measured when a person takes a lie detector test, and it is likely that a cat can tell someone is lying (even though they may not care).

We may think of olfaction as a useful tool for hunting, but hearing, vision, and touch supply most of the information needed for catching food. The sense of smell is more useful as a channel of communication between cats. The most familiar example of this is the unfortunate (to us) habit of spraying urine to mark territory. I frequently treat indoor cats that have become anxious or changed their behavior for no apparent reason, and my first suspicion is always that some aggressive outdoor cat is urine-marking on the outside of the house, the feline equivalent of threatening graffiti. Sometimes the indoor cat will attempt to put up its own "no trespassing" sign by spraying urine on vertical surfaces within the home. This is only the most obvious form of olfactory communication, and there is no doubt that many other smell messages are used, but we are too "nose blind" to even notice. When I come home from a day at my veterinary clinic, I know that my cats can tell that I have handled a dozen other strange felines, but they usually seem to forgive any offensive smells that I bring with me.

Not all chemical signals arrive by way of the nose. Cats are particularly sensitive to pheromones, airborne chemicals that are sensed by a tiny patch of receptors in the on the roof of the mouth called the vomeronasal gland. Cats generally prefer not to breathe through their mouths (which causes distress when a cat's nostrils are congested by a minor respiratory virus), but they will open their mouth to draw air across the vomeronasal gland. If the smell is particularly interesting, the cat may exhibit a unique behavior called "flehmen", in which the upper lip is raised in an Elvis-like sneer to more effectively sample the air. When an odor is sensed by the vomeronasal organ the message is sent directly to the emotional center of the brain in the amygdala. Other parts of the brain are not consciously aware of the smell, but the emotional impact is direct and powerful. Most pheromones have to do with sexual activity, but one of the pheromones has found use in reducing anxiety, aggression, and urine marking. Glands along the cat's cheeks normally produce a "friendly pheromone" called Feline Facial Pheromone; part of the reason that your cat rubs the side of his face along your leg is to mark you as a friend. A synthetic version of this pheromone is available from veterinarians and pet stores as a spray or as a plug-in diffusor[4]. When a new cat is introduced to a cat household, owners may use the diffusor to add a friendly "everybody get along" ambience to the environment. If a cat has been spraying urine in the house, the area of marking may be sprayed lightly with the pheromone; the theory is that the cat who feels stressed or threatened will approach the area to spray, but will be interrupted by the happy, relaxing effect caused by the pheromone. In my experience, about half of the cats will experience the intended effect of the spray, while the other half will show no response. Curiously, one cat behavior specialist observed that the cats who respond to facial pheromone products are the same ones that enjoy the scent of catnip. Contrary to rumors, cats that roll around in an ecstatic trance from contact with catnip are not high, but just experiencing a very pleasurable feeling triggered by the smell. Although the similarity to the pheromone reaction suggests a direct link, catnip is smelled by nose, not sensed by the vomeronasal organ. Not all cats respond to catnip, but the reaction in those cats that do is intense, although short-lived.

The sense of smell cannot be discussed without mentioning taste. As in humans, much of what we label as taste is actually a set of crude sensations from a small group of "taste buds", which is then elaborated by the smells that accompany the food. The feline sense of taste might seem a little unfamiliar to us: Humans have taste buds for sweet, salty, sour, bitter, and umami (savory), while the cat can taste salty, bitter, acid, and water. The ability to actively taste water is curious, but since water is a precious commodity to the desert cat, there is value in the ability to taste the presence of moisture. Cats are thought to have little or no ability to taste sweets, evidence that cats are not adapted to high carbohydrate foods. It is harder to explain the recent discovery that cats have seven different types of bitter taste receptors[5]. Since most bitter compounds are found in plants, biologists have assumed that bitter taste buds help grazing animals avoid toxic plants, a function that should not be useful to the carnivorous cat. Bitter tastes may serve a function in detecting toxins in the bloodstream or the microbes that cause respiratory disease. Alternatively, bitter tastes may be used to choose plants to ingest for "self-medication". Naturalists have long suspected that some wild animals selectively chew on certain plants to eliminate worms or repel parasites, and the combination of bitter taste receptors could potentially allow the cat to pick just the right herb to nibble when intestinal distress occurs. Whatever the function, sensitivity to bitter taste may account for some of the famously finicky eating behaviors of cats.

One curious aspect of feline taste is that humans and dogs find higher fat foods more palatable, while cats (despite being adapted for a high-fat diet and having the ability to smell, but not taste, fat) are not influenced by fat content. Instead, cats are attracted to foods that taste tangy and acidic. When cat food manufacturers discovered this in the 1980's, they started spraying phosphoric acid on the surface of their dry cat foods to make them more palatable. One of the unintended (but beneficial) effects of this addition was to create a more acid urine, which reduces the tendency to develop urinary blockages caused by mineral crystals. Urinary obstruction still occurs, but far less frequently than before acids were used as flavor enhancers. One might think from the above discussion that the combination of vision, touch, smell, and taste are adequate to provide cats with sensory superpowers, but the sense of hearing may be the cat's most impressive ability.

Humans can hear sound frequencies up to 20,000Hz, while dogs are famous for their ability to hear sounds up to 40,000Hz, inaudible to our ears. Cats can hear sounds into the 50-65,000Hz range, a sea of squeaks, whistles, and vibrations that we can hardly imagine. The extremely sensitive hearing of cats is further enhanced by large ears that can be directed to gather and concentrate sound like a parabolic sound collector. With all this high-fidelity audio equipment, cats are able to hear a ten octave range and discern differences of one tenth of a tone, the envy of any human musician. In addition, the brain can locate a sound within three inches from a yard away by comparing the sounds reaching the two ears. The mice and birds that interest the cat produce noises that are quiet and high-pitched, but cats are well equipped to hear the faint chirping of a mouse in its den or the rustle of a leaf disturbed by a bird foraging for seeds. We can only guess how much distress cats experience from the constant barrage of man-made sounds in our home. We occasionally see a cat with behavior changes related to unnatural sounds produced by the circuitry in a clock radio or a fluorescent light fixture.

Not all unnatural sounds are objectionable, however. The effect of music on cats has been studied, and some cats seem to enjoy a little Mozart. In general, feline stress hormones decrease when listening to classical music, while stress increases when listening to heavy metal. It may not just be a matter of a cultured ear; the high-pitched overtones of violins and flutes may be more enjoyable than the lower-pitched distortion of guitar "power chords" or the rumble of a heavy electric bass. Some researchers have even created "music for cats" by extracting the frequencies and patterns that elicit the most favorable response and combining these to create easy listening music for cats.

When cats combine their high-definition hearing ability with their vision, touch, smell, and taste, they can sense the world in ways that humans cannot imagine. When Oscar, the nursing home cat, cuddled up to patients in their final hours, it revealed more than the exquisite combination of senses that allowed him to know when death was approaching. From my conversations with cat owners, I think it is likely that most cats are able to sense human health and emotions, even if we don't know how. One of my own cats, a beautiful long-haired tortoiseshell Siamese cross named Blue Eyes, could sense when either of our children was ill. We called her our "nurse cat", because she would stay on our daughter's bed all day long when she had a virus, or with our son when he was recovering from oral surgery. The moment that "her patient" felt better, she would resume her normal routine around the house. Similar stories have been shared by many cat owners. The question is not "how do they know", but "why do some cats feel an obligation to watch over us?" The feline senses allow the cat to know us, but the social bond that they form with us may be even more mysterious.

Chapter 3: SECRET SENSES

We know a lot about the cat's five major senses, at least from a scientific perspective, but we still have a hard time understanding how cats know so much. Every cat owner has stories of their cat's mysterious behavior.

When I was in veterinary school at Washington State University, my wife and I lived in "married student housing", a tiny two-room temporary unit constructed during the Second World War but still in use for impoverished student couples. Casey Cat, the first of our own pets, shared our cozy housing. Casey Cat was a beautiful black and white cat with soft medium-length hair and an expressive voice that could be alternately intimate and endearing or demanding and impatient. Our unit was located next to a large overgrown field, and when the harsh weather of the Eastern Washington Palouse Country mellowed she spent most days exploring this grassy domain. The one thing that Casey Cat did not like was the six-hour car ride that was required when we drove to Seattle for school breaks and holidays. No matter what we did, she would meow plaintively, and then angrily, for the entire trip. Eventually she had had enough, and on the morning of one of our trips she disappeared into her outdoor sanctuary. No amount of calling or searching was successful, and eventually we gave up and asked our neighbors to watch for her and put some food out until we returned. From then on, she disappeared any time that we had a travel plans. We tried to keep our trips a secret from Casey Cat; we would not pack a suitcase or turn down the oil heater in the living room until we had her safely in her carrier. But somehow she always anticipated our plans. We could never figure out how she knew when we planned a drive; we would act nonchalant, not even mentioning our travel plans when she was in the house. But somehow she knew, and Casey Cat would always disappear just before our trips. This is the sort of thing that makes people believe in feline ESP.

Cat owners always wonder if their kitty has some special powers, and in a sense, they do.

We suspected that Casey Cat read something into our body language, something that we could not consciously hide. Many cat owners have experienced this phenomenon. Even the cat that will eagerly allow itself to be picked up for attention will run for its favorite hiding spot if the person even thinks about getting out the cat carrier for a trip to the veterinary hospital. No matter how much we ignore the cat as we walk across the room, the cat will give us sudden glance that says "I know what you are up to!" and disappear. Sensitivity to body language isn't mysterious, but cats have an uncanny ability to read intentions, a power that is essential to survival in the wild.

Cats are also keenly aware of their own bodies. Extraordinary balance is required when a cat walks along the top of a narrow fence or makes a graceful leap to a narrow shelf five feet from the kitchen floor. This physical prowess combines two secret senses: Balance relies on the vestibular system, a partnership between the inner ear and the adjacent brain, while proprioception uses nerves throughout the body to provide information about the position of the body and limbs. The input from these two systems is sent to the cerebellum, a wrinkled nerve center nestled where the brain meets the spinal cord. The cerebellum has been thought of mainly as a place for physical coordination, but more recent evidence suggests that it plays an important part in cognition. As Scott McCredie details in his book "Balance: In Search of the Lost Sense"[G], humans with impaired balance have problems with math and other "higher" thinking. Perhaps this confirms the idea of the "wisdom of the body", something that cats would understand.

The function of these balance system can be tested with the age-old demonstration of holding a cat upside down above a soft surface and dropping it. Cats will indeed land on their feet. Most of the time. Take my word for it and don't actually do this to your cat.

Some cats are born without the ability to balance and coordinate their movements. Feline Distemper Virus (the feline form of Parvovirus) has become rare since vaccines controlled the infection in the 1960's, although it is still common in feral cat populations. When kittens are exposed to this virus just before birth, they may not become ill (with symptoms of intense diarrhea, vomiting, and death) if the mother carries partial immunity. But the virus can sneak into the fetal brain during a critical stage of development and prevent the cerebellum from developing normally. These kittens can grow up healthy, but with no sense of balance at all. Despite their disability (or perhaps because of it), these erratic little balls of fur are endearingly cute and sociable. One of the professors at Washington State University researched this condition (called Cerebellar Hypoplasia), and he ended up with dozens of affected kittens, mostly donated by local farmers whose farm cats were never vaccinated. Any time a visitor walked in to the professor's lab they would be mobbed by kittens who wobbled and stumbled over to greet any newcomer. One of the characteristics of cerebellar balance problems is that the harder the kitten tries, the worse its coordination becomes, so the kittens' enthusiasm made them fall over in a slapstick frenzy. These kittens grew up to be happy adults, but they would never develop the secret senses of balance and proprioception. These kittens eventually found homes that accepted their disabilities and wobbled through life in their own way.

Time passes in minutes, days, and seasons. Every organism finds its own way to adapt to these rhythms, and as with everything else, cats are acutely in tune their surroundings. Anyone who has delayed their cat's breakfast for fifteen minutes knows the indignation and the feline look that says "You're late!" Cats appear to have an internal clock that tells them when their owner should be awake and when they will arrive home from work, when the food dish will be offered and when it is time for the 10 AM nap. Like clockwork, owners tell me. When my clients assert that their cat knows what time it is to the minute, I am curious: Is there an internal clock that keeps track of the hour, or does the cat pick up on other cues to figure out when to expect events in "human time". I sometimes ask cat owners: "When the clock changes to Daylight Savings Time, does your cat wake you up at the 'real' time, or does it adjust to the new time?" In some cases, people tell me that their cat maintains the "real time", only gradually adjusting their activities to Daylight Savings. However, more commonly the cat owner will tell me that their cat immediately shifts to Daylight Savings Time, which suggests that the cat is gathering other cues from its environment. Perhaps a neighbor drives off to work every morning at twenty minutes before the cat's owner usually awakes, providing an audible frame of reference. Cats have inscrutable ways of collecting information to keep their lives on schedule. It does appear that cats have an acute sense of time, whether it is biologic or gathered from other cues, and they like it when things happen at predictable times. I encourage people to give in to the feline rituals that make life orderly; a kitty treat and grooming session at 8 PM each evening gives a reassuring contour to the day for both the cat and its person. We might all benefit from some pleasant scheduled activity.

Time passes in daily cycles, but also in the changing of the seasons. Seasonal cycles of the brain and body have been well studied, and in most species they are driven by changes in photoperiod, the relative length of daylight and darkness. One might think that living indoors under artificial light would eliminate the ability to adjust to the cycles of sunlight, but even exposure to a small patch of sunlight through a window can override the effect of room light. As with everything biological, reality is more complicated than we think. The hours of sunlight change as the earth circles the sun throughout the year, but the intensity of sun's light also varies with the angle of the earth's tilt. When the sun's angle is lower during the winter months the light received by our eyes is more polarized, telling our brain that it must be winter.

It is natural for life to slow down in the winter, a time of dormancy and scarcity, so curtailing normal activities and spending more time sleeping can be beneficial. But life goes on in our busy world, and people who suffer from Seasonal Affective Disorder (SAD, or winter depression) can suffer genuine distress. It isn't just that we are lazy and unmotivated during the winter; many of our physiologic processes slow down as well, which may cause a worsening of chronic health conditions. People who work at nursing homes tell me that many of their frail elderly survive until just after the winter holidays, and then deaths are a daily occurrence. Winter is hard on people. If anything, cats are more attuned to the seasons than humans, and they show predictable changes.

The waning hours of daylight in the autumn can cause visible changes in our cats, although we usually don't notice if our cat is less active or declines to go outside for its normal rounds. A seasonal weight gain of up to 10% is not uncommon as the body stores fat for a lean winter; the extra pounds will hopefully disappear by the following summer. Although veterinarians don't use the label of SAD, every winter I see several cats that show alarming changes in behavior and activity during the time of the shortest days. Owners will report that their cat is acting lethargic and uninterested in normal activities. If everything appears normal after a complete examination and blood tests, we come to the conclusion that the cat suffers from some sort of winter depression. Fortunately, most of these cats return to their normal selves once the days start to lengthen.

As soon as the daylight hours start to lengthen noticeably in February, every unspayed female will come into heat, timing the birth of kittens for the late spring season of abundance. Even spayed females and neutered males become restless in the spring as their brains and hormones are stimulated by the primordial urges of "spring fever".

People are naturally curious about the feline ability to sense the unseen, but scientists are reluctant to stake their careers on investigations of extra-sensory perceptions.

Well-documented anecdotes about cats' ability to find their way home from miles away have spawned theories that center on the earth's magnetic field. A magnetic sense of direction is well documented in many wild animals[1]; birds follow the earth's magnetic force in their migrations, and sea turtles use faint magnetic lines in the sea floor to find their way back to the beach where they were born. Even cows standing in a pasture often align themselves toward the North Pole, so it would not be surprising if cats could read the magnetic map written on the earth's surface. If this is true, we might wonder about the effects of living in our houses that are awash in artificial electromagnetic forces.

The ability of animals to predict earthquakes have been legendary, although the results of scientific investigations have been mixed. As with everything else, it is possible that cats might know that an earthquake is coming but they may not show any evidence of concern. Various explanations have been suggested, including acoustic waves and vibrations, electrical/magnetic changes, or emissions of charged aerosols or ultra-infrared light. These theories have been difficult to test, since cats rarely give any warning that the earth is about to shake, even if they know.

We may prefer to let cats have their mystery and not try to explain it too deeply. Many people feel that cats have true paranormal abilities, able to predict the future and respond psychically to the distress of their owner from across the country. These unexplained perceptions have fueled the feline association with the paranormal. The Middle Ages were hard on both cats and witches, but many of these beliefs persist, albeit in more tolerant guises. The Internet, our own form of a magic, all-knowing ether, has no shortage of information about the occult. One website, www.witcheslore.com, states (apparently seriously) that "The witch is able to telepathically communicate with her cat familiar and has trained her cat to be on the alert for earthly visitors and ghosts, and spirits, the cat also alerts the witch to people who are good or bad". (Apparently cats are not likely to alert their witches to poor punctuation.) We seem to have developed a tolerance for alternative spirituality and the possibility of unseen powers, although I have a sense that there aren't as many "true" believers as "wouldn't it be cool if.." believers. But if personal auras, chakras, chi, and energy fields exist, we like to think that cats can see these things. Perhaps that would explain some of the mysterious behaviors of our household companions. Maybe cats can even see our souls.

Chapter 4: NOTHING MORE THAN FELINES

When Jason came home from work on Tuesday he was greeted with a shocking surprise. As he walked past the coffee table in his living room, he was attacked by his normally docile calico cat. Patches lived a quiet life as an indoor cat and she had never been aggressive toward Jason before, but this time it was serious. Patches was all teeth and claws as Jason tried to push her away from him with a couch pillow. She kept coming at him, and eventually Jason had to close himself in the bathroom to avoid being mauled. For two hours he was trapped by his cat, who suddenly seemed possessed with hatred for him. That night he closed his bedroom door, prompted by visions of nocturnal murder by his feline fatale.

The next morning, Patches seemed to be her normal self, but Jason brought her to the clinic to find out what might be wrong with her. A thorough neurologic exam revealed nothing out of the ordinary, but we discussed various health issues that could cause such sudden aggressive behavior. In the end I told him that this was most likely a delayed emotional response to something upsetting, and I suggested that he look for clues.

Tuesdays were the day that his housekeeper came by to tidy up the house, so Jason asked her if she had noticed anything unusual. "Well, your cat was sleeping on the coffee table", she answered, "and suddenly there was a terrible sound of dogs fighting next door. I went out and yelled at them to stop it, and when I came back inside your cat had disappeared under the bed in the guest room. I thought that she was scared, so I just left her alone." This seemed to explain Patches' frantic state of mind, but Jason still couldn't understand why his cat would take it out on him.

Because cats evolved to live life on the edge, their emotions are exaggerated. Feelings may remain hidden only to be revealed in stress-related disease, or they may explode into a sudden unexpected outburst. In order to understand the power of the cat's feelings, we need to consider the underlying brain anatomy and chemistry that drives emotion.

The senses gather information from the cat's surroundings and send it to the brain. Deep within the brain, the first stops are the hippocampus and the amygdala, where connections are made between a stimulus and a feeling. The smell of a freshly opened can of food is linked to the sensation of hunger being satisfied, the sight of a fleeing mouse is associated with the predatory urge, and the sound of thunder is tied to a sensation of fear. The amygdala serves as the command center for mobilizing emergency action, whether it is to run away, leap after a fleeing rodent, or rub affectionately against its owners legs. The emotional center has a threshold and once this emotional level is exceeded, action follows.

As the amygdala is unleashing an emotional response, it also sends a report to the frontal cortex of the brain so that the situation can be evaluated more fully. The executive centers in the cortex may decide, based on past experience, that there is no threat and order the amygdala to stand down. But this advise-and-consent order comes after the fact, when adrenaline is already coursing through the bloodstream. The blood pressure is soaring, the blood sugar is surging, and the heart is pounding. The adrenal glands follow quickly with a release of cortisol, creating a euphoric sensation and blocking the pain and inflammation that may result from the oncoming emergency. Because cats have a very robust emotional response, it can be difficult to rein it in once the "red button" has been pushed. This intense reaction is an essential part of the feline adaptation for living on the edge.

The rush of pure emotion isn't necessarily unpleasant to the cat. In fact, it seems that some cats enjoy the visceral rush of an emotional response. Many cat owners are familiar with the feline behavior that I call "seeing spacemen": The cat may be calmly walking across the room, when suddenly it's back arches, it's hair stands on end, and it races down the hall as if being chased by invisible demons. Moments later it will stop and calmly groom itself. It is my impression that these cats are actually imagining some fictitious scenario that activates an emotional reaction, just to give their emergency system a workout. In this way it may be like the radio that broadcasts a long tone, followed by "This has been a test of the Emergency Broadcast System. If there had been an actual emergency you would be instructed to get the hell out of town."

The aftermath of the feline emotional response may be rewarding, like the bungee-jumper who gushes breathlessly "That was so great!"—after being pulled back up onto the bridge from which she has just jumped. Cats seem to vary in their need for this rush of emotion. Some cats are "adrenaline junkies", and they may create a crisis just to get the feeling. When two familiar cats with adjoining territories engage in a hissing match it often seems like they aren't really serious about their aggressive threats. They will stand face to face with ears pulled back and teeth exposed, hissing and growling furiously. But in many cases the cats already know their territorial boundaries, making the standoff an unnecessary show of force. Instead of taking action (as they would against a strange intruder), each cat eventually turns and leaves the scene, like a duel of honor in which each person discharges their weapon and, point made, retires to the local tavern to luxuriate in the after-a-crisis feeling with his friends. A short emergency feels great after it is over, and sometimes it is worth creating the drama just for the feeling of tension and release.

But not all cats are "adrenaline junkies". Some are "scaredy cats" that seem to find the feeling of emotional stimulation decidedly unpleasant. As human caretakers we need to recognize when our kitty just doesn't need more excitement in its life. Some of these crisis-averse cats are happiest within their own tiny comfort zone of a single room, retreating under the bed every time a stranger visits the house. These cats may be outgoing, curious, and exploratory when their world is calm, but they avoid situations that trigger strong feelings.

The effects of emotional arousal and stress intersect, but they are not necessarily the same thing. In part this relates to how long the excitement lasts, and whether the cat seems to thrive on or wither from the after-glow of a sudden emotional burst. The duration of the stimulation determines whether it becomes a chronic distressing force or an exciting punctuation in an otherwise placid existence. Much of the stress that causes feline health and emotional problems gives no outward sign of excitement; like the old adage, "still waters run deep". The apparently calm cat that is subjected to change over which it has no control may suffer more than the cat that suddenly bites the hand that annoys it.

One of the most paradoxical feline behaviors that I hear from cat owners involves what we call "petting aggression". An affectionate cat sits in the lap of its favorite human, purring contentedly. The person complies with the cat's wishes by stroking its fur gently. The cat clearly enjoys the contact, rubbing against the outstretched hand and rolling on its side ecstatically, begging for more. But when the petting continues, the cat suddenly grabs the person's hand with its paws and sinks its teeth into the human flesh, and then runs off. What happened?

The answer lies in emotional arousal. In most cats there is a certain threshold of emotional arousal that triggers an aggressive response. It doesn't seem to matter whether the cause of heightened feelings is something scary, like a sudden noise, or whether it is something pleasant, such as an enjoyable petting session. Once emotional stimuli combine to exceed the cat's threshold, then aggression is almost automatic. Any retribution made by the injured and betrayed human simply makes it worse: shoving the cat off your lap or remonstrating sternly "You know better than that!" in a loud voice simply adds fuel to the emotional bonfire that was ignited by the pleasure of physical contact.

When I am questioned by distraught owners that have been attacked for giving their pet affection, I teach them how to look for the signs of emotional arousal. Every cat has its "tell", some sign that emotions are reaching a full boil. The objective is to recognize when this threshold is near and put an end to the petting session gently and calmly. Most often this means that the person needs to stand up slowly, allowing the cat to slide down to the floor gently, and simply walk away for a few minutes.

Years ago I watched a video of a hand-raised tiger at a game farm where wild animals were trained for movies. As the camera-person and the animal trainer (who had raised the tiger from a cub and clearly had a close and loving relationship with the animal) walked around the ranch-like grounds, the trainer engaged the full-grown tiger in one of its favorite games. The big cat obviously loved it, growing more animated as its handler affectionately pushed the cat's shoulder and the tiger leaned into the contact. Suddenly, the trainer casually spoke to the camera-person: "Look at what he is doing right there with his ears. He is loving our game, but if I keep playing like this for another thirty seconds he will attack me." The trainer then proceeded to demonstrate his technique for lowering his tiger's emotional level. First he stopped and looked away, talking constantly in a low, soothing voice. The tiger's ears stopped their restless movement. Then the trainer took slow small steps forward, avoiding eye contact or touching, while continuing his quiet murmuring. After five minutes the tiger relaxed visibly. At that point the trainer resumed his brisk walk, touching his tiger playfully at intervals. "Now he is fine. I know his signs, and the only way that I can live with him safely is to bring him back down before he erupts." This video demonstration demonstrated the same reaction that can cause a cat to hurt the person that they love.

Most occasions when the cat's emotions spill over into aggression are not caused by pleasant sensations like petting or play. Usually the cat has a reason, but the recipient of the cat's anger is not the one who caused the reaction. Cats are famous for what we call "displaced aggression".

If one of the cats in the household on the receiving end of an unpleasant encounter with a rival, it is likely to take it out on the next cat that crosses its path. It is an unwritten law that "If something makes a cat angry, then someone must pay!" And that someone is often not the one who caused the reaction. This is what happened to Jason when his cat Patches forced him to take refuge in the bathroom. The terrifying din of angry dogs outside raised her emotional level to the point where it needed to be discharged, and "someone must pay." Jason suffered the fury because he was the next person that Patches encountered. Even though Patches seemed to have gotten over the episode by the next day, Jason noticed for the rest of the week that his cat would give him a little hiss when he walked by the coffee table. Apparently Patches still considered that the "scene of the crime", and she relived a little of her trauma every time the association was made. Just in case, Jason moved the coffee table into another room for a few weeks. Because you never really know what a cat is thinking.

Fear and anger are considered different emotions, with different pathways in the brain. In cats, these feelings are usually found together, mixed in different proportions: A frightening episode might cause a timid cat to hide under the bed from fear, but if you reach under to bring him out you will likely receive an angry reception. Sometimes an angry reaction may be triggered by something less than fear, such as the annoyance of being forced out of a favorite chair. We would do well to recognize that a nervous cat is only a small step away from being an angry cat.

Sadness is the third of the classic five emotions, and the hardest to detect in cats. We can assume that they feel melancholy, but we are unable to read their body language well enough to be empathetic. Grief is a special form of sadness, one that cats definitely experience. Wildlife biologists bear witness to heart-wrenching scenes of grief in wild animals: The moose that languishes by its dead calf for days, the elephant herd that circles a deceased member in obvious distress, and even the reaction of magpies in what can only be called bird funerals. In cats, grief takes the form of a sickness behavior with lethargy and loss of appetite. I have often seen cat patients who are brought in after their housemate (either human or feline) has died, and the owner is concerned about their pet's behavior. Sometimes the stress of losing a companion pushes the cat into a serious illness, and the reaction is more than just depression. In many cases the reaction is mainly emotional, but these cats suffer as well. Fortunately, time heals, and by the end of a month the sadness of the loss fades, although the memories last.

There can hardly be grief without love. Some would say that love is a strictly human emotion, but we can closely correlate the feelings of love with rises in oxytocin, the bonding hormone. When biologists look at relationships in mammals they find that oxytocin rises when animals form close bonds, such as in mated pairs or friendships. In dogs, physical closeness and prolonged eye contact raise oxytocin levels in both the dog and its owner, proof that we love our pets and that they return the emotion. Oxytocin levels in cats have received less attention, but we can be confident that their apparent aloofness conceals a bond of love.

The last of the five emotions is joy. We understand some of the chemistry of this emotion in humans, a surge of dopamine in specific parts of the brain. But what does this look like in a cat? Most dog owners can clearly tell when their dog experiences joy, with enthusiastic leaping, vigorous tail-wagging, and a happy facial expression. As I try to imagine what joy is like to a cat, I come back to the idea of an animal born to live on the edge, using its supersenses and agile movement to claim dominion over its environment. Relationships enhance the joyous feeling, sharing the moment in some cat-like way.

Many years ago I witnessed a scene that suggests what joy must be like. Thousands of runners were crowded into the wide street between Seattle's old Kingdome stadium and a tall condominium complex. As I waited with the other runners for the start of the annual Seafair 5K, I noticed that everyone was looking up at the condo building. Spectators lined the balconies, and on the fifth floor a cat was perched confidently on a narrow balcony railing. The runners below held their breath, expecting to see the cat fall to its death. The cat seemed to play to the tension in the crowd as it calmly walked back and forth on the railing. As if it was showing off, the cat proceeded to move from its own railing to the adjoining balcony, which required wrapping its body around eight inches of intervening wall where there was no railing. The cat repeated the feat four times, a feline circus act with an anxious audience of spectators holding their breath. This is what I imagine joy is like to a cat; exulting in the use of its powers and controlling the reactions of those around it, the ultimate and literal expression of living on the edge.

Chapter 5: A SENSE OF PLACE

The skies were overcast on moving day, a persistent drizzle falling as John and Rebecca loaded their household belongings into a rented truck. The couple was only moving five miles away to a more spacious house on Seattle's Eastside, but they worried about how Gandalf, their tabby-colored Maine Coon Cat, would handle the move. Gandalf had been confined to the laundry room during the moving operation to prevent his escape in the confusion as boxes and furniture were being loaded. Finally the packing was complete, Gandalf was coaxed into his carrier for the short trip to the new house, and the door to the old place was closed.

At the new house, John and Rebecca prepared a comfortable place in the spare bedroom so that Gandalf could have an area all to himself while he adjusted to the new house. Everything went well, so during the second week he was allowed the freedom of the house, quickly adapting to new locations for the litter box and food dishes. All went well until the third week, when the front door was accidentally left open, and Gandalf was gone.

John drove around the neighborhood, trying to catch a glimpse of his cat's round face and tufted ears. Rebecca put up flyers: "Lost Cat: Doesn't answer to anything, but you can call him Gandalf and return him to us". After two weeks, however, there was no sign of Gandalf and hope gave way to a sense of loss.

Later that month, Rebecca received a call from one of her old neighbors. "Why didn't you take your cat with you? We see him nearly every day since you moved, sitting on your back porch. We feel bad for him, so we leave him a little food, but he must be missing you." Sure enough, when Rebecca drove back to her old house Gandalf walked up and nonchalantly rubbed against her leg in his customary greeting. It was shortly after this adventure that Gandalf's owners called me in desperation: "How can we convince our cat to accept the new house so that he doesn't run back to his old home?"

This story is common, but the question is hard to answer. Cats love their family, it is true; but they are tethered to their territory by even stronger bonds. This is one more example of the feline legacy of living on the edge. The only security is the security of place. Even for the pampered house cat, home is where the food supply is guaranteed, the smells are familiar, the litter box is in just the right spot, and where treaties have been signed with the neighboring feline population. Change is dangerous, and the only protection lies in the security of a familiar and well-controlled environment.

What would make the ideal place for a cat to live? If there was an online real estate listing service for cats, the checklist for the cat's dream home might run something like this:

- Dining establishment is convenient, nearby, and open all night.
- Elimination facilities are private and well maintained.
- Cozy and spacious rooms offer good insulation and light.
- Located in a nice quiet neighborhood; sounds of traffic and dogs are limited.
- Neighbor cats are friendly, neutered, and have no territorial claims over the house and yard.
- Comfortable resting spots, preferably elevated, are plentiful and available for sleeping and watching. Secret hiding places offer opportunity to get away from it all.
- House smells fresh, with no lingering odors (or fleas) from previous residents.

- Surroundings are well-appointed with familiar furnishings and decor.
- All of your favorite people live there, ready to satisfy your every whim.

In our civilized urban world humans seem to have lost the sense of belonging to a place, but this need is still a part of the feline psyche. We can't appreciate how a cat experiences life without considering the place where their life happens. There is no place like home.

Homeland security ranks high on the daily concerns of any cat, whether it patrols an extensive outdoor territory or shares a city apartment with two other cats. Many of the objectionable behaviors of house cats have their roots in territorial marking. Some of these methods of staking claim to a place are familiar, but others may be more hidden. The important thing is that nothing a cat does is accidental; life on the edge doesn't allow the luxury of wasted effort. For the cat that is allowed to go outside, establishing territorial boundaries is a priority. If a cat moves into a new neighborhood, it is likely that other outside cats in the area have already annexed these outdoor spaces into their own territory, and they will resent any intrusion by a newcomer. In my experience, territorial disputes between resident cats in suburban areas are resolved without bodily harm. The cat-next-door may simply allow its own territory to shrink as the new cat patrols its yard and plants its flag by urinating and scratching on strategic landmarks. At some point the cats will cross paths, and a hissing match may ensue. Usually both antagonists will eventually back away, satisfied that their negotiation has set the boundaries. But stray cats, particularly non-neutered males, present a tougher problem for the newcomer. These bad boys are full of hormonally-driven aggression, and usually lay claim to larger areas of turf. Stray male cats seem to prefer fighting to negotiation, and establishing a secure territory often results in injury to the new cat.

My sister-in-law's cat discovered a novel way to establish territory. Their family moved frequently, changing houses every year, and RJ made every move along with the rest of his family. This gray and white male kitty didn't have an assertive personality, but he did like to spend part of his day enjoying sunshine and the smell of the grass and garden. The family also included Kelly, a muscular little black terrier-mix dog, which the cat tolerated. A pattern developed at each new house in which RJ would venture outside only when the dog was also present in the yard. After a month of this RJ apparently felt that his borders had been secured, and he would feel safe enjoying the yard by himself. Interestingly, no other cats were ever observed near the yard, and Kelly showed no overt protective tendency toward the cat. But by the fifth time this pattern was repeated it was clear that RJ had learned to establish his claim to territory with the help of his own personal canine bodyguard.

Just as with international diplomacy, feline interactions can be subtle, agreements established by back channels and gracious posturing. This might involve two cats simply watching each other from a distance until there is an unspoken re-drawing of the property line. Urination and defecation help to provide olfactory title to any disputed land. And the act of patrolling the borders is often sufficient, even without any physical encounters.

One of my own cats took a particularly gentlemanly approach to territorial defense, especially in his later years. Snowy had lived in our house for eighteen years, ever since early kittenhood. He liked to sun himself on a second-story deck at the back of our house where he could survey the lower parts of the yard a hundred feet distant. Occasionally some other cat would wander into the lower section of the yard to investigate something and Snowy would suddenly notice the intruder. He would rise, stretch indolently a few times, and march resolutely down the deck stairs to defend his territory and his honor. Snowy had never been a fighter (he suffered only one cat bite during his two decades as an indoor/outdoor cat), and it appeared that the neighborhood cats must have respected him. But they didn't fear him. As Snowy marched down toward the distant parts of the yard to enforce his borders, the intruder would often loiter around, investigating the weeds around our garden shed. If the stranger didn't start to leave as he approached, Snowy would simply walk slower and slower, but with the same air of authority. It was as if he would tolerate no territorial disrespect, but he would allow the interloper ample opportunity to make the right choice and leave on his own. As soon as the other cat left, Snowy would hurry down to the area where he had seen the cat, scrape the ground with his hind paws, and leave a few drops of urine as a reminder that he still owned this corner of the earth.

For the inside cat, territory is more complicated. This creates situations that are stressful to both the cat and its owner. While it might seem that the cat that never leaves the safety of its own home would have little to worry about, the opposite is often true. The indoor cat may feel like a captive, under constant threat from outside.

Cat owners often consult me about cats that have developed troublesome behaviors like urine marking or scratching furniture, or about pets that suffer from stress-related diseases like Inflammatory Bowel Disease. The person will insist that there has been no stressful change in the cat's life to trigger the problem. The most common source of threat for the indoor cat is the presence of a new member of the surrounding feline community, particularly a homeless stray. Although people usually tell me that they have not seen any unfamiliar cats hanging around, the indoor cat would tell a different story. Since one of a cat's favorite activities is to stare out the window to monitor every detail of life on the outside, cats certainly know more about neighborhood animal activity than we do. With exquisite sensitivity to sounds, the cat may even hear the rustling footsteps of a neighbor cat, which seem silent to us. And above all, the smells left by a wandering stray are overwhelmingly apparent to the cat who is a prisoner behind his window. The most serious intrusions of unwanted visitors happen in the middle of the night, when stray cats are emboldened by the cover of darkness and the lack of human activity. When I explain this to a cat owner, I can often sense that my client has doubts about my narrative of their house under siege by unfriendly felines. At that point I propose an unusual investigative technique: "When you go home today, walk around the outside of your house and sniff. If there is a seriously unfriendly cat in the area, you will probably notice the smell of cat urine, particularly near the doors or under the windows. Your cat certainly knows the meaning of those scent marks". This suggestion is often met with an expression of mixed interest, disgust, and social aversion ("I am not going to sniff my house! What would the neighbors think?"). But with surprising frequency cat owners return and report that they discovered the acrid scent of tom-cat urine on the exterior of the house, a message of threat and territorial conquest to the cat that is confined indoors. In order to put the owners in the mindset of their cat, I suggest that they "imagine that you got up this morning and found your front door tagged with threatening graffiti. You may not have seen or heard anything, but it would certainly make you feel anxious!"

Since territorial security is central to the cat's peace of mind and quality of life, unwelcome visiting cats can be discouraged in several ways. Urine marking is the most serious intrusion and homeowners can hose off the areas on the outside of the house where stray cats are most likely to leave their urine marks: under the windows, near the sliding glass patio doors, and by the garage and front doors. It is said that all members of the cat family dislike the smell of citrus fruits (African explorers reportedly sprinkled bits of orange peel around their camp to keep lions away, a seemingly flimsy defense), so an orange-scented air freshener spray can be used to "counter-mark" areas where stray cats may approach the house. I have laced my own front garden with pieces of orange peels to keep nocturnal visitors from defecating in my planted areas, and it has been effective.

The protected zone around the house can also be enforced with a motion-activated device. The one I use is a small inexpensive plastic unit that produces an annoying alarm-clock sound for thirty seconds any time an animal breaks the invisible beam. Other products are available that turn on sprinklers when motion is sensed nearby. Often these deterrents are only needed for a few days, since stray cats will learn the unpleasant consequences after one or two experiences.

It should be noted that not all visitations by outside cats are unwelcome or threatening. One of my own indoor cats developed a remarkable friendship with a cat that lived two houses away. Every few days a short-haired tortoiseshell kitty would show up under our front window, chittering and meowing in a way that even a human could understand as "come out and play!" Only one of the four cats in our house

would respond. Puffy was our female seal-point Himalayan who had been a show cat until she developed annoying
urinary behaviors and her previous owner became frustrated and gave her up. When Puffy heard the sounds of her
visitor, she would run to the front window and engage in
friendly conversation with the other cat. These two cats
never met directly, but it was obvious that these visits were
friendly and pleasurable to both cats.

There is much more than security that makes a house a
home. Cat psychologists refer to the enhancement of the
cat's living space by the term "environmental enrichment",
and creating the perfect vibe for the individual cat adds
pleasure and contentment. We will discuss enrichment at
length in Chapter 11.

A house is not a feline home without a selection of comfortable resting spots. Cats will find their own favorite
place on the couches and beds, but many cats prefer an elevated place where they can rest "above it all". The carpeted
"cat trees" sold in pet stores are a good start, but with a little imagination other areas on bookcases, tall furniture, or
loft-like ledges can be made accessible to the cat, allowing
both a feeling of security and control—an area where the
cat can nap and not be bothered by household activities. In
one house, the office/den featured bookcases extending

from floor to ceiling. The books and knick-knacks were removed from one of the shelves just above human eye level and the owner fashioned a cat-friendly ladder with wide carpeted steps, placed at an angled slope that allowed his cat to scamper easily up to her private perch on the shelf. During the evening hours when her owner worked at his desk, his cat Bebop could always be found watching from her favorite spot.

Another feature valued by the truly contented cat is a good observation spot from which the cat's kingdom can be surveyed. One of the most deeply feline traits is the need to keep an eye on their surroundings. Wildlife biologists have found that any habitat where mountain lions, bob cats, or other wild felines live will feature at least one good lookout spot where the animal can watch for danger, learn the movement patterns of local prey animals, track territorial invasion, and stay in touch with changing weather conditions. We occasionally read about a case in which a displaced mountain lion wanders into an area inhabited by people, raising a panic of alarm in a suburban neighborhood. Wildlife officials are called in, and the animal is darted with a tranquilizer gun, thrown in a truck, driven to some far-off area in the mountains, and released. We would like to think that the wild animal will naturally settle into a new location. After all, food, water, and shelter are abundant, why wouldn't the cat feel right at home? But if the new area lacks a good vantage point from which to observe the surroundings, the cat will move on, looking for a home with a broad vista.

Fortunately, an observation spot is one feline necessity that we can provide in our homes. The elevated resting spot is a good place from which to watch the indoor environment. A perch by a window provides even more rewards. The movement of birds, bugs, and other small creatures satisfies the predatory interests of the cat, but in some cases owners feel that stimulating the urge to hunt without the ability to do so may create frustration. For some cats this may be true, but studies suggest that wild cats track the movement of every small animal within their range, so that when hunger strikes it knows right where to find its next meal. Watching potential prey may be more like counting potential resources than "kitty pornography"; rather than stimulating an unattainable desire, watching birds flitting through the bushes may be entertaining and provide a feeling a plenty, of a rich environment where prey is plentiful.

The dark side of providing an outdoor view is that the sight of intruding cats can create anxiety. Some cats may become stressed, surveying their yard with anxious concern rather than tranquil contentment. When this is the case, the steps described to discourage roaming cats should be considered. As long as stray cats are not disturbing the peace, most cats enjoy a room with a view.

Not all of the qualities of the feline dream home are visible. If we shared the cat's acute hearing, we might find that the air is full of sounds that bombard the senses with noise. Most people have experienced the feeling of walking into a room where the television is turned up so loud that our nerves are on edge; "Could you turn that down!", we plead with our teenager. It is likely that cats are more volume-sensitive than we are, but if they find something unpleasant they are usually quite capable of retreating to another room There are other sounds that our human ears cannot hear in our house. When electronic appliances are engineered to operate quietly, this is often done not by eliminating clicks, hums, and vibrations, but by hiding these distracting noises above and below our range of hearing. The cat senses the ultrasonic shrill of the crystal in our clock radio and the infrasonic vibrations of the fan motor in our heat pump, and these could easily stress the cat by making constant demands on the cat's nervous system. And let's not forget sounds from outside; I have had several cats who developed stress-related vomiting problems when roofers were working on a house across the street, or dogs in the neighborhood were barking constantly. We don't often consider the effect that our noisy high-tech homes inflict on our cats, but we should think about what noise pollution is doing to our cats—and ourselves!

Even more than sound it is smell that makes the feline home. Every place that a cat sleeps is permeated with its personal scent, an olfactory sign of ownership. When moving to a new home, it is helpful to bring familiar odors from the old house: Clothing worn by the owner, blankets that the cat used for bedding, and even potted houseplants can provide known smells to make the cat feel at home. Cats usually customize their home with their personal scent, rubbing their sides and face along surfaces to give the house a lived-in ambience.

The pheromone diffusers mentioned in Chapter 2 provide a sense of calm and belonging. In my own clinic, we used a pheromone diffuser in the feline treatment area and kennel at all times; any little bit of comfort that we can provide seems worthwhile. The smell of lavender has been shown to decrease stress-related responses as well.

There are undoubtedly smells that create stress, but often we don't know enough to avoid them. Odors from strange cats are one obvious negative, as are citrus scents.

Flowery odors used as deodorants in scented cat litters and some other household products seem to be annoying enough that many cats avoid the litter pan if it smells like a French garden. The best we can do is to be observant and try to eliminate odors that the cat avoids. For example, after cleaning the bathroom with bleach and strong disinfectants, it is helpful to rinse the disinfected surfaces and air the room out before opening it back up to the cat. Your cat may not show it, but it will appreciate the effort.

When more than one cat lives in the same house, they need to negotiate a way to share the space. Cats often divide up their territories, even inside the house. Male cats tend to claim more of the house than females, mirroring the behavior of wild cats, in which females will establish adjacent territories and males claim much larger territories that overlap several female domains. Cats usually work out their own arrangements, but often the process is invisible to humans. Behaviorists have been surprised by how complicated these household relationships can be.

In one study[1], eleven cats of varying ages and genders were moved into an old house. Observers recorded where each cat slept, rested, and groomed. Elaborate time-sharing patterns emerged. Initially, each cat occupied a limited area in the house, but these household ranges gradually expanded. Eventually a pattern emerged in which each cat chose a small number of favorite sleeping spots. These areas were also used by other cats, but each set of locations was used only by members of its own distinct group of cats. These time-share groups tended to consist of a few males or a group in which a female had a maternal relationship with the others (either her grown kittens or other compatible cats that were "adopted" by the female). Cats did not tend to use these resting spots at the same time, but even when the spot was vacant members of other groups would not be found there. There seemed to be no competition or aggression involved with maintaining the "ownership" of these favored resting spots, but cats can always manage to make their wants known. In my own house I witnessed an interesting variation on this ownership of special spots. At the time our household included three of our own cats, each with such different personalities that they didn't interact much. We were familiar with the favorite sleeping spot of the oldest male, Snowy. But when our son came home from college for the summer he brought along his cat, a large sleek tabby male named Apollo. All of the cats coexisted peacefully, but we noticed that Snowy's favorite spots were now occupied by Apollo. At first we thought that the outsider simply chose the best seat in the house, but when Snowy spent a few days at our veterinary clinic, Apollo abandoned the spots that previously belonged to Snowy. Apparently Apollo's appropriation of those areas was simply a way to send a message that he could do as he wanted, even if he was an outsider. As soon as Snowy returned after a few days at the hospital, Apollo could be found right back on Snowy's favorite spots. Nothing that cats do is ever by accident.

One curious phenomenon described by many cat owners (and witnessed in another of my own cats) is that some cats may shrink their comfort zone down to a very small area: the top of the refrigerator, the space under a raised fireplace hearth, or a small corner of the den. What is unclear is whether the cat is being intimidated by other household cats and feels that it can only hold claim to a small space, or whether the cat is trying to avoid some unpleasant stimulus and stays in a tiny area where it won't be bothered. When cats choose an elevated area (such as the top of a chest of drawers), it sometimes turns out that there are fleas in the carpet and the cat has learned to avoid the painful bites by heading for higher ground. There may also be areas that are safe from unpleasant sounds or vibrations of which we are not aware. But in many cases it appears that the cat has decided that it simply doesn't want to venture away from its small comfort zone except to attend to the necessities of eating and eliminating. What I have observed in these cases (including my strange cat Jazzmine, who lived under the fireplace hearth) is that these cats seem happy in their tiny home area. Better to feel safe and secure, even in six square feet, than to be insecure in a larger area.

When cat owners seek practical advice about getting a cat adjusted to a new house, there are a few simple guidelines. The most effective technique is to confine the cat to a single room for one week, providing all of the amenities that make the cat feel secure and well-provisioned. Ample food and water (including extra-palatable food choices, such as canned food along with dry) should be provided, along with a litter pan in a spot where the cat can use it without feeling cornered or exposed. If the cat is already bonded to the people (as when moving to a new house), old clothes or blankets permeated with the owner's scent provide a sense of home. Only after a week should the cat be allowed out to explore the rest of its new house, and only after a month should it be allowed outside (if an indoor/outdoor lifestyle is the chosen option). In this way the levels of stress hormones have a chance to subside, allowing the cat's natural curiosity to take over. Then the exploration and claiming of a new environment will become a pleasure.

Even with this routine of gradual adjustment to a new living space, it is common for a cat to disappear the first time it gets out of the house (either with or without permission). The despondent cat owner will often call up to report that their cat has disappeared, and they feel that they will never see it again. My prediction is that within thirty-six hours their kitty will show up, nonchalantly demanding a meal and its favorite sleeping spot. It seems to be standard protocol for the cat that takes its first jaunt out-of-doors to hunker down in a secret hiding place near the house where it can see and hear everything in the area without being found (owners always claim that they have searched everywhere; I don't know how these cats manage to make themselves invisible, but I am convinced that they are hiding within thirty feet of the house). As soon as the cat has taken a full inventory of the surroundings and all of the nearby activities, it will return.

Most cats adjust to a new territory after only a few stressful weeks. Gandalf, the kitty we met at the beginning of this chapter, was the exception in returning to his old haunts. Was there something about his old house that drew him back irresistibly? Or was there some unseen aspect of the new house that made it seem like an undesirable place to live? After Rebecca drove across town and retrieved Gandalf, she once more confined him to his private room for a week. She provided all of his favorite foods and soft music, and when he was once more allowed out into the rest of the house, he strutted around with an attitude that spoke clearly: "This place is mine".

Chapter 6:   WHAT'S FOR DINNER?

What do cats really want for dinner? One adventurous
group of researchers wanted to find out what happened
when cats ate as they did when the domestic cat's natural
habitat was the barn and dinner was whatever scurried
around in the hayloft. Cats eat rodents, reasoned the scientists, so they threw dead rats in a blender to produce a
crunchy puree of natural cat food. Apparently the cats
thought this rat-atoulle was delicious, and they seemed
healthier and more energetic after their diet change. When
faced with many of the chronic problems of the thoroughly
modern cat, it may be helpful to think of how they lived in
the wild.

One effect of living on the edge is that cats have much
more demanding nutritional needs than dogs or humans.
We know that ancestral cats hunt birds and mice, but we
don't appreciate that cats are trapped by the demands of
being an "obligate carnivore". The resourceful stray dog
can get by on just about anything it finds; a half loaf of old
bread from a garbage can, an apple found under a neglected

tree, or a road-kill possum. But a cat is a cat, and if it cannot find fresh meat it will eventually perish. We have been slow to learn this nutritional truth as cats have moved into our houses and away from the small edible animals outside.

Using the ancestral feline diet of rodents as a model for improved nutrition could also be misleading. While it can be argued whether human Neanderthals actually ate Paleo, it is likely that they exercised hard and lived only about three decades. Eating for longevity was not an evolutionary prerequisite. Similarly, wild members of the cat family are more likely to die young than to fall victim to slowly developing nutritional imbalances; one study compared the diseases of inside and outside cats and found an average life expectancy of fifteen years for the inside cats, while the lifespan of the cats in the great outdoors was only three years. But even though the "good old days" don't always tell us how to eat for longevity, there is value in examining the ancestral diet to see what hints it gives us.

Nutritionists have their own ways of looking at food. The traditional approach of nutritional research involves feeding a particular nutrient, such as protein or vitamin D, in different amounts to determine the "minimum daily requirement" for the substance. Once the needs for protein, fat, vitamins, and minerals are calculated, producing a cat food becomes a simple exercise in mathematics. But the devil is in the details, and simplified assumptions have resulted in some misguided feeding practices. One of these painful lessons in feline nutrition claimed one of my own cats.

When cats suffer from heart disease, it almost always involves the muscle of the heart, rather than the defective valves that cause most canine heart problems. There are two forms: Hypertrophic Cardiomyopathy, in which the heart muscle becomes so thickened that the chambers of the heart cannot fill completely, and its opposite, Dilated Cardiomyopathy, in which the muscle wall of the heart becomes so thin that it can't contract with sufficient strength to push blood around the body. During the 1970's and 80's, the dilated form of heart disease was the most common, and we saw at least one cat every month that would suddenly become weak and collapse, usually dying before we could help—and there was no effective treatment. A clue to this devastating disease came when a stubborn cat owner refused to believe that nothing could be done for her beloved cat with dilated cardiomyopathy. Her cat was already being treated for blindness at the University of California at Davis Veterinary School and at that time it was already known that a deficiency of the amino acid taurine could cause degeneration of the retina. This cat's owner believed that her cat's heart problem simply must be related to the taurine-deficient vision problem. Cardiologists insisted that this wasn't the case, but some cat owners can be downright pushy when it comes to their kitties. Measurements of taurine in the blood were indeed low in this cat, which prompted an urgent study of the link between taurine deficiency and the heart. This became a top-secret investigation, because researchers realized that if they reported that cat food with insufficient taurine was killing cats then cat food manufacturers would face a firestorm of litigation. After only a few months this study was prematurely terminated when it was obvious that taurine deficiency was indeed the culprit. Larger amounts of taurine were required to keep the heart muscle functioning in some cats, and even a slight deficiency could cause fatal heart disease. The announcement of this breakthrough was as dramatic as the research. One Wednesday night I was attending a scheduled lecture by Dr. Mark Kittleson, the cardiologist from UC Davis, when he announced that he would be cutting his scheduled lecture on heart disease short to "share a little something new we have found". The research paper that broke the news about taurine and cardiomyopathy was to be published the following day in the prestigious journal

Science[1], and he figured that he could let us in on the news a day early. The cats that we had seen dying in our practices simply needed higher levels of taurine in the diet, he told us, and the heart could repair itself.

It isn't often that medical progress leaps forward in such dramatic fashion, and every veterinarian in the lecture hall sat in stunned silence. This discovery struck me particularly hard; one of my own cats had collapsed and died from dilated cardiomyopathy the previous week. If this lecture had been one week earlier, my cat Miranda would likely have lived to tell the story. Cat food manufacturers immediately added generous amounts of taurine to their cat foods (I suspect that the cat food companies had gotten advance notice so that they could claim that they were already on top of it), and dilated cardiomyopathy in cats became a thing of the past.

The taurine story is only one in a series of discoveries that points up the truth that cats are not merely small dogs nor can we extrapolate their needs from human nutrition. People and dogs can produce their own taurine from other amino acids and don't require it in their diets. The cat body is a demanding and specialized high-performance system that demands more than just calories and vitamins to stay well. This has created some controversy and uncertainty when it comes to feeding cats.

The idea of feeding a diet of pre-made dry kibble harkens all the way back to James Pratt, an American living in London in the 1800's He noticed that the limey sailors fed their sea biscuits to their dogs, and it inspired him to create a crunchy portable food for dogs. Cats were still expected to fend for themselves, and even on shipboard there was no shortage of rats and mice. It wasn't until the 1930's that Americans could buy packaged (canned) food for their cats. Dry cat food was born out of necessity when World War II created a shortage of tin for cat food cans, and a new form of food was developed that could be stored and sold in paper containers. This new form of food required new ingredients: A dry pelleted food could not be produced unless it contained at least 40% carbohydrate, in the form of starch. Initially the source of carbohydrates was grains and corn, but now that "grain-free" has become a marketing slogan in human foods, feline kibble producers have turned to other carbohydrates, such as potatoes, casaba root, or tapioca. Newer foods may be grain free, but they still use carbohydrates as a major ingredient.

We should have been paying more attention to the cat's carnivorous needs with the taurine/heart disease problem. It turns out that mice, birds, and other small prey are a very good source of taurine (the name of this amino acid suggests it is found in bull meat, although I don't picture many cats taking down a big bovine), so there was no pressure for the cat's ancestors to make their own taurine. Cats were meant to thrive on a carnivorous diet, without the carbohydrates that have been added to modern cat kibble.

The most convincing evidence that a new approach to feeding cats is overdue comes from research into diabetes mellitus, a disease that consumes a large share of human healthcare efforts. Diabetes was once rare in cats, but no longer; at least once a week we see a cat in our clinic that is losing weight, drinking excessively, and suffering from nerve problems or urinary infections. These cats are almost always older than five years and weigh over fifteen pounds. There are several types of diabetes: Type 1 diabetes is seen in dogs, an immune disease that destroys the pancreatic cells that produce insulin. Large or obese cats are susceptible to Type 2 diabetes, in which excess body fat and stress hormones block the effects of insulin so that sugar cannot be burned up by the body. Most cats over fifteen pounds could be labelled "pre-diabetic" and may be pushed over the edge into full-blown diabetes by the slightest stress.

Even at this pre-diabetic stage, cats simply don't feel as well as they deserve to.

At Colorado State University, Dr. Debra Greco was studying feline diabetes when she made an accidental discovery. The trace elements vanadium and chromium were thought to improve the function of the body's own insulin, and when Dr. Greco supplemented one group of diabetic cats with vanadium, their blood sugar improved significantly. This seemed to offer a new tool to help the fat, sugary feline feel better. To her credit, Dr. Greco started to wonder about these results. In order to medicate the cats with vanadium, she had been mixing it with canned food, although all of the cats were normally fed dry kibble. What if the beneficial effect was due to feeding canned food, rather than the vanadium? When she repeated the study but fed the canned food without vanadium, the results were the same: the majority of cats showed an improved blood sugar and they felt better[2]. Apparently the canned food, low in carbohydrates, was responsible for the improvement.

Intriguing as these findings were, Dr. Greco took it one step further. Since most diabetic cats are overweight, she wondered if fat cats that were not diabetic would benefit from a canned-food-only diet. It turned out that most obese cats shed their extra pounds with this simple low-carbohydrate diet change. The university had some funds that had been earmarked for whole-body scans, so Dr. Greco used this opportunity to see how these cats' bodies had changed with the canned diet. As suspected, the cats on canned food (a canned kitten food product was chosen for its extra high protein content) lost fat, gained muscle, and their metabolism improved. Some of the overweight cats in the study did not lose any pounds, but even these cats converted from flabby tabbies to fit felines. When canned food replaced dry, the essential change was an increase in protein and a decrease in carbohydrates. Canned foods usually contain almost no carbohydrate, while kibble requires at least 40% carbohydrate to form it into a dry pellet.

The no-carb approach to feline nutrition has been labelled the Catkins Diet (apologies to Dr. Atkins and his famous diet for humans). A diet based on protein and fat actually makes more sense for a feline carnivore than it does for an omnivorous human evolved for a diet rich in fruits and roots.

Since Dr. Greco's groundbreaking work on diabetes, the no-carb diet has been shown to be the most effective means of weight control. For many cats, dry foods and the carbohydrates they contain are satisfactory, but for many carbo-hydrate-intolerant cats the carbs contribute to obesity.

As veterinarians, we tend to try everything out on our own animals (and sometimes on ourselves) when we hear of a new concept. Shortly after Dr. Greco started advocating for low-carb diets, I had the perfect opportunity.

Mugsy was one of a litter of newborn kittens that were dropped off on my clinic doorstep in a paper bag one chilly May morning. Once we warmed the kittens and fed them they all came around, and were raised by hand at our clinic. When my daughter left for college a few months later she took a short-haired female with "lynx point" Siamese coloring and a long-haired tabby male. The male kitten was half the size of his littermates, so she named him Mugsy, after the diminutive NBA basketball player Mugsy Bogues, whose 5'4" stature made him a shrub among the redwoods on the basketball court.

As often happens with an abnormally small kitten, Mugsy continued to grow, even after his littermates attained their full size. And he kept growing. By the time he was four years old, the scale groaned at 22# when Mugsy was placed on it. This cat was a case of diabetes waiting to happen, so when Dr. Greco's research suggested a no-carb approach I knew just the cat to try it on. My daughter and her fiancé had just graduated from college, and she asked if I could keep Mugsy and his sister while they took a lengthy post-college road trip. I had six months to see what a new diet could do for an obese cat.

Mugsy and his sister Juno started a simple no-carb diet: Each morning and evening they shared a 7.5oz can of kitten food. Sometimes a spoonful of canned pumpkin would be added for additional fiber. Both cats seemed to enjoy their new food, but I was surprised that neither cat seemed hungry during the day; in fact, even if I offered a snack at noon they didn't seem interested.

By the time my daughter had returned from her long road trip, Mugsy had shrunk from twenty-two pounds to fourteen, while his sister had gained from eight pounds to nine. Most importantly, the energy and activity level of both cats had doubled, and their rambunctious games of chase shook the house.

This first experience with carbohydrate reduction has been repeated hundreds of times in my patients. Although I still counsel portion control, low fat, and high fiber, these approaches rarely work. I offer the canned-food-only approach when weight loss is critical to the cat's health. The protein-fat-and-fiber diet may be the best way to give our cats the feel-good energy of their wild cousins.

This ancestral approach to diet is not universally accepted. Veterinary nutritionists have long insisted that "a calorie is a calorie", whether it comes from protein, fat, or carbohydrate. There are several reasons why this may be overly simplistic. When carbohydrates are ingested and digested, the blood sugar rises rapidly and the pancreas secretes insulin to drive the glucose into cells. As the blood sugar drops the brain sends out signals that more food is needed to bring the glucose back up. The end result is the storage of more body fat, causing the cells to become less sensitive to insulin. Cats are poorly adapted to riding this blood-sugar roller-coaster. On the other hand, protein releases glucose slowly as it is digested and the change happens so gradually that the pancreas only has to trickle insulin into the bloodstream to handle it. The blood glucose stays at a relatively constant level, suppressing the hunger response. This is the classic description of why carbohydrates increase obesity and help cause diabetes.

Recent research suggests that there may be another reason that carbohydrates and obesity are linked. The intestine provides a home to bacteria, billions of organisms and thousands of different species. This "microbiome" regulates a variety of processes throughout the body. We will explore the microbiome and its effect on the cat's well-being in Chapter 8 but here it will suffice to point out that the population of microorganisms in the intestine is a reflection of the food that we feed. As a broad generalization (at least in carnivores), harmful bacteria are lazy, and they are better suited to the easy energy provided by carbohydrates. Healthier types of bacteria tend to adapt to living on proteins and fats. Even fiber, although it provides no energy that can be absorbed by the body, provides food for beneficial intestinal bacteria.

Recent studies in a variety of species have shown that the particular types of bacteria in the intestine can promote either obesity or weight loss. No single species of microbe can regulate body weight; in one mouse study[3], a cocktail of 54 strains of probiotic bacteria promoted healthy weight loss, but a mixture of only 39 strains failed to show this effect. The most startling finding in this and succeeding studies was that the bacteria actually turned the animals' own weight-regulating genes on and off. The invisible hand on the controls of many body functions belongs not to the cat itself, but to the microscopic residents of the intestine. And what we feed these tiny tyrants makes a big difference.

The beneficial effects of a diet closer to the wild are evident, but how can we improve our cat's quality of life with this information?

One of the trends in recent years has been to feed a raw diet. After all, the wild cat doesn't process it's food or cook it; it goes straight from burrow to breakfast. Since this is the case, wouldn't it be better to feed food raw? A raucous controversy surrounds this issue, fed by emotion, well-intentioned internet opinion, and a substantial helping of moral indignation directed toward pet food mega-corporations and modern life in general. While there is an element of truth in the raw diet concept, there are some problems.

Studies have defined two main hazards of raw diets. The first is that—well, they are raw. Cats are not immune to harmful bacteria that can be found in meat-producing animals. Campylobacter is the most common food-borne germ that causes diarrhea humans. Hand washing is suggested after handling raw chicken, since it commonly carries the bacteria. In the veterinary clinic it is not uncommon to diagnose cats with diarrhea caused by Campylobacter, although the source is rarely known. Salmonella is the most notorious of pathogens found in uncooked meats, and it also presents a clear and present danger to cats fed raw food.

The argument that cats have always been exposed to harmful bacteria in their food does not take into account that meat raising practices have changed dramatically in the past fifty years. The crowding of cage-raised chickens and feedlot cattle has increased the levels of bacterial contamination of meat a thousand-fold. This is not your grandmother's free-range farm food. Most raw meat available in grocery stores presents a potential source of disease if not cooked thoroughly, and that goes for cats and dogs as well as humans.

Although raw-food enthusiasts have suggested that cats are naturally resistant to the bacteria that commonly are found in raw meat, our experience with bacterial diarrhea argues otherwise. In fact, there is a natural raw source of intestinal infections; up to 70% of small wild birds carry Salmonella, and cats occasionally develop "songbird fever" from consuming the birds that they catch.

The second danger of raw diets is that they may be nutritionally unbalanced. Cats have very exacting nutritional requirements and there is little room for error when putting together a feline diet. Even an experienced nutritionist may have difficulty finding the optimal combination of ingredients to keep a cat healthy and happy. While it is true that cats in their natural state eat meat, there is more than meat in a meal of mice and birds. Connective tissue, internal organs, and bits of bone provide completely different nutrients than muscle tissue. In the first half of the 20th century nutritional bone disease was common because many cats were fed strictly meat scraps. The proper ratio of calcium to phosphorus in a cat's diet is 2.1:1, but meat has a ratio closer to 1:10, with far too much phosphorus for the amount of calcium. Excessive phosphorus pushes calcium out of the body and bones, resulting in bones that are soft, achy, and easily fractured. Mineral imbalances exist in many of the homemade diet recipes that are found on the internet.

One more food issue deserves mention. At one time fish was commonly used as cat food, and it was associated with several health problems. Some cats developed crusty bumps on their skin, which veterinarians often called "fish eater's skin". It may be that fish was unfairly blamed, but there are some cats that do seem to react badly to fish foods. One explanation is that the fish used in cat food is not processed into cans immediately, and it undergoes deterioration that produces histamine and causes an allergic-like reaction in the skin. Some cats may be allergic to the fish itself, and some may simply have chemical reaction to the histamine. Since the types of fish used in cat food are usually bottom fish, there is also concern about the mercury level that could be present. In addition, fish foods are high in magnesium, which may contribute to the formation of irritating urinary stones and crystals. Although our concepts of bladder disease have changed, avoiding excess magnesium is still a wise choice. The popularity of fish-based cat foods has declined, and that is probably a good thing.

Finding the perfect diet for our cat's well-being is no simple task, and it is worthwhile to feed diets that have been vetted by the pet food company nutritionists, despite the fact that they may have conflicting interests and that our knowledge of cat nutrition is still not complete.

As we have seen, diabetes and dilated cardiomyopathy have their roots in nutrition, but there are many other examples of the close link between food and wellness. As we will discuss in future chapters, both urinary and intestinal health are strongly affected by what is in the food dish. Most importantly, the needs of one particular cat may not be the same as for other cats. Even before the taurine content of commercial foods was beefed up, the great majority of cats did not develop heart disease. The active nine pound cat is unlikely to develop diabetes, even when it eats a carb-rich dry food. And the cat that enjoys a rewarding and stress-free home life may not develop bladder disease, not matter what it eats. Diet, genetics, and lifestyle interact in a complex blend to support the good life.

Chapter 7: OLD AND NEW WAYS

There was a time when lions and men lived in the Kalahari desert with mutual respect and toleration. The Ju/wa bushmen had inhabited the harsh wilderness of central Africa for thousands of years, sharing the position of top predator with the lions that fed on the wildebeest and antelope that lived there. Lions were aware of the bushmen and the Ju/wasi kept a close eye on the big cats, but lion attacks on humans were rare.

Elizabeth Marshall Thomas, who grew up in Africa, describes the ancestral respect that these two groups shared prior to the 1950's[A]. But then the local government evicted the aboriginal people of the Kalahari, leaving the lions to live alone in the wilderness. In the 1980's, humans started to once again visit the area that had been the exclusive domain of lion prides for thirty years, but mutual respect and forbearance were a thing of the past. Lion attacks now occurred with dangerous frequency, creating a tense atmosphere for both humans and lions. Ms. Thomas uses this example to support her contention that members of the cat family establish local cultures, similar to the human cultures that define distinct groups of people around the world.

Some philosophers and scientists resist using the word "culture" when discussing animal behavior. Anthropologists define culture as "the sum total of ways of living built up by a group (of human beings) and transmitted from one generation to another." A broader definition includes transmission of behaviors within a group of individuals, such as the fads shared by human teenagers. Cat behavior is complex, but can we consider feline behavior a form of culture?

Life on the edge can be challenging, and cats need to be flexible when adapting to change. Not every new behavior is helpful, but a willingness to try new things without abandoning successful behaviors is a strategy that has helped cats survive and thrive.

One of my favorite things about cats is that they seem to invent new behaviors out of thin air. Dogs have a lot of interesting behaviors, but they tend to be the same ones; dogs do what other dogs typically do. But nearly every day a cat owner will tell me about some quirky habit that their cat does, some behavior that I have never heard of before. One cat collected stray pennies (and only pennies) and stashed them in a special spot under the sofa (the owners only discovered the hiding place when they got new furniture). Another cat arranged rats that it killed in neat rows on the walkway outside the house. My own cat Ania has a special routine when my father-in-law visits; she likes to dip her paw gingerly into his coffee and lick the drops from her toes. She doesn't do this with anyone else and my father-in-law doesn't encourage it, but it must mean something to Ania. For any given unusual action a variety of sensible explanations could be concocted, but the uniqueness of each behavior suggests that cats often like to try things out, and in some cases these become entrenched as regular habits.

We can glimpse how feline culture works by considering how cats drink. One of my regular questions is to ask cat owners is "Is he drinking water?". Clients always assure me that their cat is drinking, but when I ask "Does he drinks out of a cat dish on the floor?" many cat owners become vague. When pressed they will often divulge the quirky little secrets of their cat's drinking preferences. One older man finally confessed, "Well, Athena meows in a certain way to tell me that she wants me to fill her special orange glass 1/2 inch from the top and put it on the nightstand by my bed". One cat I know insists that her owner/servant put one ice cube in her water dish and stir it for a few seconds. My daughter's cat Mugsy accompanies anyone who goes into the bathroom and then he leaps up to the sink for a drink. But rather than just pouring a little water in the bottom of the sink (a favorite of many cats), he wants a slow drip, about one drop a second. He licks the water as it collects in the bottom of the sink. Drops continue to fall on his head while he is licking the moisture in the basin, but this is part of the game; the moment the tap is turned off, he won't drink the water that remains in the sink.

Each of these unique habits is completely individual; other cats in the same house normally don't participate, so these routines might not qualify as cat culture. Unless the humans are included in the social group, that is. The common denominator of many of these drinking games is that the cat is able to beg, cajole, or threaten the person into performing a role in the activity. Since other humans tend to provide the requested service, it can become part of a family culture as more people reinforce the behavior. It is my impression that cats develop these routines because they like "teaching" their humans to perform a requested action. Dog owners brag "Look what I trained Fido to do!"; one can almost hear cats claiming "Look what I trained my people to do!"

Quirky behaviors aside, there are a lot of interesting aspects to water drinking in cats. Having evolved as desert animals, healthy cats have a number of mechanisms that allow them to subsist with very little water intake. Although water should always be available, most cats don't really drink very much. In fact, if an owner tells me that they notice their cat drinking regularly from its normal water bowl, I start to wonder if the cat might have some health problem that causes it to drink excessively. Cats are able to concentrate their urine by reabsorbing water from the urine as it passes through the kidneys, so that waste products can be eliminated with minimal loss of precious water. This hyper-concentration makes cats very resistant to urinary tract infections, although the increased concentration of urine minerals can lead to bladder stones.

Cats have an additional way to produce water internally. A unique feline pathway for metabolizing protein releases a molecule of water for every protein molecule broken down. With these water-conserving and water-producing tricks, healthy cats can (if needed) get by on very little water. It is said that lions in the Kalahari can live through the dry season without drinking water as long as they have sufficient fresh meat to fill their bellies.

Although drinking water from a dish may be somewhat optional, there are many times when more water consumption is desirable. This has led to some clever ways to encourage cats to drink more water.

As the fascination with dripping sinks and draining bathtubs suggests, running water may be more enticing than water that sits motionless in a dish. This has led to the invention of water dishes that recirculate water over a spillway with a small pump to create motion.

A pair of my own cats, nearly identical gray-and-buff twins, found a glass bowl with a cut-glass pattern on the sides irresistible. The bowl was originally purchased as a table decoration with three red floating candles that bobbed on the water. Even with the candles floating on the surface Muffy and Roxy would drink the bowl dry every day. It seemed that sun coming in our dining room window sparkled on the patterned glass in the side of the bowl, giving the water a flickering illusion of movement. Certainly a preference for moving water makes sense for the wild cat; as every hiker knows, a running stream is cleaner and safer to drink from than a stagnant pond. When we want to increase a cat's water intake for medical reasons, we often suggest trying a circulating water dish. But of course, cats are never that simple.

To investigate the preference for flowing water, experimenters in one study[1] provided circulating water dishes to half of their cat subjects, and normal dishes to the other half. After several weeks the dishes were switched to the opposite type for comparison. Careful measurements of the water consumed were made every day, and on average the cats drank the same amount regardless of which dish was used. But closer analysis told a more complicated story: Half of the cats clearly preferred the moving water to drink, while the other half showed a strong preference for water that stayed still. Even in water drinking habits, cats are individuals; they each like what they like.

Another strategy that has been used to encourage more fluid intake is to add water to the food, or replace dry food with canned food, which is 80% water. This is traditionally suggested by veterinarians, but it appears that cats have roughly the same total water intake whether their food is dry or wet. Cats fed dry food simply drink more water to make up the difference[2]. As discussed in the previous chapter, there are nutritional benefits to feeding canned food, but the high water content is apparently not as much of a benefit as has been thought.

If culture is a set of behaviors that are passed from individual to individual resulting in a localized "way of doing things", it might be argued that idiosyncrasies like water drinking habits aren't culture but simply quirks of the individual that are not usually shared with other cats in the household. However, sociologists Janet and Steven Alger provide a different perspective on the culture question. In their book "Cat Culture: The Social World of a Cat Shelter"[D] the Algers studied the interaction of cats and their caretakers in a unique shelter in England where as many as sixty stray cats roamed uncaged in four small rooms, interacting freely with a parade of other cats that ranged from feral strays to abandoned pets. These authors promote the sociologist's perspective that culture, individual behavior, and even the concept of self-awareness are only constructed within a social framework. They observe that many of the unique behaviors of their shelter cats are the result of give-and-take interactions that include other cats as well as the humans that provide them food, shelter, and affection. When my daughter's cat Mugsy would leap to the bathroom counter and demand that someone would turn the faucet to a slow drip, a unique ritual was born of the feline request and human response (only hair-splitters would use the term "manipulation"). By including human participants, it is evident that this becomes a cultural exchange, whether other cats opt to participate or not. The human/feline inter-action creates another way of doing things for the cat.

We may not recognize shared influence between cats because other cats in a group may observe the way another cat does something, but choose not to follow suit. Other times a behavior can be contagious. At one time my own home hosted six cats of varying backgrounds, from a semi-feral female to a spoiled Himalayan show cat that was banned from its previous home for inappropriate urination. At the time, we fed a dry cat food that was formed in the shape of an "X", provided in two large dishes. This worked out well for several years, until one of the cats de-cided that it would not eat any crunchie that had one corner of the "X" broken off. All of the other cats gradually adopted this prejudice against broken kibble. It took some time for us to finally realize that none of the cats was eating the food, despite the cat dishes being full to the brim. Upon close examination, every piece of food in the bowl had a broken part, and none of the six cats was willing to eat them. As soon as the broken bits were emptied and re-placed by fresh, fully-formed crunchies, the cats all ate rav-enously. This pattern of rejecting damaged kibble persist-ed, even after we tried a fresh bag of the same food. Even-tually we were forced to switch to a food that came in a rounded shape, with no corners to break off. This prejudice spread rapidly among our feline household, but how this habit spread among our cats was not clear.

There are subtle ways in which information is passed from cat to cat. One fascinating example involves hunting skill in house cats. We know that an interest in hunting and the skills to support it are passed down from mother to kittens. Genetics has a part to play, and kittens born to great hunters tend to share those skills. Mother cats also school their offspring in the art of capturing prey, when possible by bringing home live mice for the kittens to practice on. But as always with cats, there is more to it. One study involved two mother cats, an experienced hunter and a cat that showed no interest in hunting. These two queens had litters at the same time and experimenters switched the litters at birth. It was not surprising that the excellent hunter's kittens turned out to be better hunters than their foster mother who had no interest in hunting. The unexpected finding was that the kittens of the non-hunting mother became excellent hunters when raised by the experienced huntress. These kittens became better hunters than their biological mother, but they also performed better than the hunter's own natural offspring. They apparently learned their craft from the experienced cat, but how? In this case, the hunt-savvy mother was not allowed any opportunity to hunt, so the kittens did not learn by observation, or by paws-on practice with real prey animals. The kittens may have learned skills from their adopted mother, but how this information was passed on is a cultural mystery.

Elizabeth Marshall Thomas provides another example of how cats are willing to modify their local customs when it came to living with other cats. She lived on a farm with a large number of cats, and a pattern developed in which her cats responded to the introduction of any new cat by moving to the outbuildings and only gradually coming back to the house once the newcomer was integrated into the social structure. But when they moved into a suburban house, the cats abandoned this culture of letting each new cat have its space. Somehow they established a different way of coexisting without physical separation, much like the cats in the Alger's crowded shelter.

If cats are capable of inventing creative new ways of doing things, why do they cling so firmly to these behaviors once they are established? If they can adapt to a changing environment by altering their habits, why are they so stressed when we move the furniture to a different spot in the living room? And if they can embrace social structures as different as the solitary territorial cat, the matriarchal clique, or the bohemian live-and-let-live lifestyle of a crowded free-range shelter, then why does the introduction of a second cat create emotional upheaval for a house cat?

Perhaps the answer lies in the way that cats evolved for life on the edge. The wild cat's world is difficult and dangerous, with little tolerance for strategies that are not tested and proven. But when situations change, a willingness to experiment may be the only hope. And if the new way of doing things is successful, the cat can once again cling tenaciously to a new normal.

Chapter 8: THE INSIDE STORY

Stepping on a damp mass that your cat has thrown up on the carpet in the middle of the night is one of the questionable perks of cat ownership. My cat Ania is currently the only cat in our house and finding a regurgitated mass of hair and food on the floor is a common occurrence. Her hair is long and black, and when she vomits we find a slimy cylinder of saliva-covered hair. We inherited Ania when she was two years old, and although she has always thrown up about once a month, she has never gone off her food. Veterinarians and cat owners alike have traditionally blamed this pattern on hairballs in the cat's stomach. Most people tell me that their pets throw up from time to time, and they are not worried about it; after all, that is what cats do, right? Wrong. Intestinal symptoms can have a profound effect on how the cat feels, and they are a signal that life is not as good as it should be.

This chapter will be devoted to the intimate workings of the feline gastrointestinal tract, so the queasy reader can skip straight to Chapter 9. However, this is something that we need to bring up (pun intended), because the digestive system has a big part to play in the cat's health and happiness. The link between the brain and the body is written in the inner workings of the mouth, stomach, and intestines. Part of what follows may seem like too much information about the workings of the largest internal organ, but if we are to understand our cats, we need to appreciate what goes on inside them.

Before proceeding into the dark depths of the feline GI tract, let's explore the connections between the intestine and brain. The symptoms of intestinal disease are sometimes obvious: Vomiting, diarrhea, poor appetite, or weight loss justify a trip to the veterinarian. But even when there are no external signs, the intestine exerts a profound influence on the sense of well-being. Mild GI cramps can cause an intermittent discomfort, rarely evident to the cat owner. More importantly, there is a neural highway that runs from the internal organs, particularly the intestine, to the brain. This nerve is given the name of the Vagus, the "wandering nerve", and it provides two-way communication between the internal organs and centers deep within the brain that provide homeostasis. The vagus nerve helps regulate the bowel, moving digested material through the intestine and squirting it with just the right enzymes and juices to turn it into absorbable nutrients. This same nerve tells our mouth when to water, our skin when to sweat, and our heart when to slow down and rest. All of this essential maintenance information is fed to areas in the brainstem so that appropriate out-going signals can be sent to make minute-to-minute adjustments to bodily functions. What is less appreciated is that the vagus nerve continues to wander up into the parts of the brain that influence mood and emotions[E].

This interaction of brain, bowel, and mood happens constantly inside all of us without our awareness. If we feel a little down or anxious and stressed for no apparent reason, the vagus may be partly to blame. And the largest amount of input to the vagus comes from the intestinal lining. A recent study[1] in mice gives a hint of why we should appreciate this body-brain link.

In 2011, John Bienenstock at McMaster University in Canada and John Cryan at University College Cork in Ireland measured how the stress hormones in mice rose with a mildly distressing test in which the mice had to walk a maze suspended over water, so that a misstep would force the mouse to swim for safety. Then the mice were fed a probiotic mixture of healthy intestinal bacteria. After being fed the probiotic for 3 weeks, the mice were again tested on the maze. The mice that received probiotics had levels of stress hormones half those of their untreated friends. How could putting new bacteria into the intestine change how the brain feels? To find out, they severed the vagus nerve connecting the intestine and the brain, and the anti-stress effect of the probiotic disappeared. This elegant experiment demonstrates that when the intestine is happy, the brain is happy.

Interestingly, the intestine also performs its own sort of thinking process. Nerve networks in the gut have millions of complex connections, and they use many of the same neurotransmitters found in the brain. Most notably, serotonin (the brain chemical associated with calmness and decreased anxiety, the target of Prozac and many other antidepressants) was first discovered in the intestine, where 90% of the body's serotonin is found. The complex workings of the intestinal nervous system and its communication with the central nervous system have led neuroscientists to nickname the intestinal nervous system "the second brain".

The two-way communication between intestine and brain goes the other way as well. The concerns of the brain have significant effects on the gut and other internal organs. But enough neuroscience for now; what does this mean for the cat?

Our perspective on "hairball vomiting" was challenged by startling study[2]. It has always been assumed that any cat that throws up once a month is a normal cat. Since the contents of the vomit often consist of a soggy mass of hair and saliva, the vomiting has been intuitively blamed on the irritating effect of hair in the stomach. Some cats throw up food occasionally, and cat owners tell me that it is because "he eats too fast", a reasonable conclusion. Ingesting grass can also be aggravating to the stomach and cause hairball-like vomiting, but grazing on grass seems to be a normal cat behavior; many people even provide special "kitty grass" in shallow trays for their inside kitty to chew on. And cats do throw it up on occasion.

Dr. Gail Nordsworthy, a respected but free-thinking cat veterinarian from Texas, started questioning our long-held assumptions about occasional vomiting. In an initial series of cases, he convinced 200 owners of cats with occasional vomiting to have intestinal biopsies done. This could have been done by inserting an endoscope through the mouth of the anesthetized cat, a relatively non-invasive procedure. But we already knew that the shallow samples taken at surgery with an endoscope fail to tell the complete story in the majority of cats. Full-thickness biopsies taken from the middle section of the intestine (along with samples of the stomach and other organs) provide much more accurate information. What Dr. Nordsworthy found with his first 200 hair-ball vomiting cats was that only two cats had a normal intestine. The other 99% of his patients (remember, these were not sick cats, just cats that threw up occasionally) at surgery had some disease process in their gut. Owners perceived the occasional depositing of food or hair on the floor as a mere annoying inconvenience, but now that we realize how even mild complaints from the intestine can affect the mood and brain's enjoyment of life we need to look in more depth and not accept even occasional vomiting. Since the original study by Dr. Nordsworthy, an additional 100 cats have been examined, with similar results.

From a science standpoint, there was a major piece of information missing in this study. All of these cats had symptoms, even though they were mild. We don't know what the biopsies from cats with no symptoms would have shown. Autopsy studies have shown that pancreatitis, which is frequently associated with intestinal disease, may be present in 16-20% of cats that have no symptoms at all. My own suspicion is that if enough normal cats were tested we might find intestinal disease in half of the cats that roam our houses with no apparent distress. Why is the domestic cat's intestine so unhappy?

When biopsies are taken from a cat with persistent vomiting, diarrhea, poor appetite, or weight loss, the most common diagnosis is Inflammatory Bowel Disease (IBD), a common irritation of the digestive system. IBD is essentially the result of the immune system overreacting to mild or imagined insults. Under the microscope the intestinal lining appears infiltrated with an excessive number of white blood cells from the immune system. There are different types of immune cells found in different flavors of IBD, but they all release irritating chemicals that damage the lining of the gut and interfere with absorption of digested nutrients. And the intestine sends its complaints up the vagus nerve to the brain, where this bad news can suck away the enjoyment of life. But most cats don't complain.

There is a metaphor that I use to help clients understand the inflamed bowel. White blood cells are the armed forces of the body, rushing into battle when a threat occurs. Imagine a village in rural France during World War II; when the Allied soldiers showed up to drive out the Nazi invaders, the villagers were delighted to greet them with hospitality and gratitude. But fast forward to several years later: The German threat had been eliminated, but many of the Allied troops were still there keeping the peace—and drinking their wine, chasing their women, and creating the annoyance that even well-meaning outsiders can bring to a peaceful town. I imagine the immune cells infiltrating the inflamed intestine as those soldiers: welcome when there is an enemy at the gates, but irritating when they don't go home after the battle is won.

Humans also have intestinal maladies similar to IBD, the most familiar of which is Crohn's Disease. People don't usually share too many details about this embarrassing source of internal discomfort but it is something that a person can't ignore. Crohn's Disease is as mysterious and intractable as the feline form of IBD, although much less common.

The most common diagnosis in Dr. Nordsworthy's cat study was IBD, but it was followed closely by a low-grade type of lymphoma. The biopsies in small-cell lymphoma look very similar to IBD, but the white blood cells that invade the intestinal lining are cancer cells rather than normal immune cells. From a practical standpoint, there is not a sharp dividing line between IBD and low-grade lymphoma; if the same biopsy sample is read by three different pathologists, it is likely that there will be disagreement about how to classify the sample. Even when the same pathologist looks at three samples from the same patient, it is common that two samples will be diagnosed as Lymphocytic Enteritis (the most common variety of IBD) but the third sample from the same cat will be labelled as lymphoma. Both of these diseases are treated similarly, but presumably the lymphoma cats will not do as well as the more benign IBD cases. There has been suspicion (although it is still controversial) that IBD may be a way-station on the path to lymphoma, which has encouraged veterinarians to be more proactive about diagnosing and treating IBD at an early stage or attempting to prevent it altogether.

More recently, veterinarians have noticed that cats with chronic pancreatitis (inflammation of the pancreas) and cholangiohepatitis (inflammation of the liver around the bile ducts) feature immune cells that look just like the cells found in the inflamed intestine. When multiple biopsies are taken, it is common to find that two or even three of these related organs are involved, which has led us to think of IBD, pancreatitis, and cholangiohepatitis as three different faces of the same over-reactive immune system. This combination has been given a new name, Triaditis. But this new label doesn't tell us anything new about why cats' react this way.

We are what we eat, the popular slogan declares, and this is especially true for the cat's exquisitely adapted digestive system. As we discussed in Chapter 6, dry foods high in carbohydrates, preservatives, and coloring agents are not ideal for the cat. There are many ingredients in commercial cat food that would be foreign to the wild cat intestine, and we know very little about how the gut reacts to these substances.. Even though scientific proof is scarce, clinical experience tells us that searching for the right food is important to intestinal health.

In some cases the cat may actually be allergic to some ingredient in the cat food, and a proper food allergy trial is in order. This involves feeding a specialized diet containing no ingredient that the cat has ever eaten. In order to be meaningful, the strict food allergy trial must be done for eight weeks, which is more than most cat owners are able to do. More commonly the problem is not an allergy, but what we call an adverse food reaction. Some aspect of the food disagrees with the digestive system; this may be some ingredient, the balance of protein/fat/carbohydrate, the cooking process, or some other factor that we have not yet discovered. Without a specific dietary culprit, searching for the right food can be a needle-in-a-dungheap proposition.

Dr. Mike Lappin is a noted feline veterinarian who teaches and does research at Colorado State University, and he tells this story of his own experience. Dr. Lappin is a world authority on cat diseases, but when he lectures he seems like the kind of regular guy that has to clean up cat puke on his floor like the rest of us. He is an entertaining speaker, with long wavy hair that has turned silver, a bit of an Oklahoma drawl, and an irrepressible sense of humor. He tells about when his mother-in-law's cat developed chronic diarrhea. This was a wonderful opportunity to impress his wife's family with his world-class expertise. When the standard treatments failed, he performed every diagnostic test that the CSU lab had to offer and collected multiple biopsies to confirm IBD. Prednisone (the first choice drug for IBD) had little effect, as did intestinal antibiotics, motility modifiers, and probiotics. His mother-in-law was not impressed that her famous veterinarian son-in-law couldn't even cure a cat with diarrhea. Dr. Lappin continued his efforts by cycling through the various prescription diet options: bland diets, high-fiber diets, food allergy diets—nothing seemed to make any difference, and he continued to endure the scorn of his mother-in-law. In frustration, he instructed her to simply try different pet store diets, starting at one end of the cat food shelves and working her down the aisle, feeding each food for two weeks before switching again. None of the foods helped, until she got to the 12th product on the shelf, and the within days the cat's stool became normal and the kitty became noticeably more playful and active. Good for the cat, not so much for Dr. Lappin's family reputation: "Why didn't you just tell me to feed that food to begin with?" was all his mother-in-law could say.

Diet is important, but so are the billions of bacteria that normally live in the intestine. Most are our friends, some not so much, but they all have a profound effect of our well-being. The bacteria living in our body outnumber our own cells, and it turns out that these microbes can turn the genes in our own cells off and on for their own benefit. We are truly not alone; as one biologist puts it, "Bacteria run the world, we just live in it." Nearly every day another study reveals some startling aspect of the relationship between the body (human, feline, or other) and the "microbiome"—the complex web of microorganisms that lives within us.

In our search for a better internal life for our feline friends, there are a few discoveries that are worth considering. As previously mentioned, mice could be made more stress-resistant by supplementing their diet with a bacterial probiotic that sends calming messages up the vagus nerve to the brain.

Ninety percent of the body's immune system lies within the gut, and intestinal bacteria play a vital role in modulating the response to invading infections. Some bacteria help by encouraging the immune system to play nice with the other cells in the body.

Even more surprising is the role that intestinal bacteria play in obesity. A number of studies (again, in rats; the time and expense of doing these studies in cats makes study impossible) have shown that the type of bacteria in our intestine can make us lean or overweight.

If the intestinal microbiome is this important, one road to internal health would seem to be probiotic supplements, but this is a complicated subject. The gut can be thought of as a rich ecosystem of interrelated bacteria, hopefully being fed by healthy nutrients and living in harmony with the intestinal lining. Just as a forest ecosystem relies on fungi to break down the soil, plants to stabilize the soil, bees to pollinate the plants, trees to create shelter and shade, birds to spread the seeds, and dung beetles to consume all of the feces produced by the deer, bear, rabbits, and mice, the intestinal "circle of life" depends upon thousands of species of intestinal bacteria contributing to the balance of the GI community. Healthy bacteria make a happy intestine, but just adding a little yogurt or a supplement of Lactobacillus is not enough to achieve the digestive good life. We don't know how to provide all of the bacteria needed for intestinal health, but giving probiotic supplements may still be a desirable thing to do. Side effects are very unlikely, and the potential health benefits are great. As more research is done, we will find better ways to influence the microbiome. For now, there are a few guidelines:

The type of bacteria included in a probiotic is important. Some species of bacteria improve stool quality, while others regulate the immune system. Certain species help disable potentially harmful microorganisms, while others aid in weight control.

Probiotic bacteria need to be given in sufficient numbers. We don't know the exact counts needed, but a good starting point is one billion organisms per day. By comparison, even a typical live culture yogurt may only contain ten million bacteria in a human-size serving.

Probiotics are living organisms, and what really counts is how many live bacteria are given in each dose. Even a good quality product with a label that claims ten billion bacteria per dose may have little effect if it is exposed to excess heat or sits on the pet store shelf for several months. Many people feel that a quality probiotic should be sold from a refrigerator, but some of the better quality products claim to have processes to keep the bacteria alive for long periods, even at room temperature.

We need to provide the right foods for these beneficial bacteria in order to help them do their jobs. If we give a supplement of billions of fiber-loving bacteria but don't feed the right kinds of fiber, it is unlikely that these good bugs will stay around for very long.

We don't know enough about the use of probiotics yet, but my recommendation to cat owners is fairly simple: Find a high quality product that contains at least a billion organisms per dose, including strains of Lactobacillus, Bifidobacterium, and/or Enterococcus; a variety of bacteria is probably a good idea. Many owners use good human products, although there are several appropriate veterinary probiotics available. Most of these products can be sprinkled on the food daily, and cats generally like the taste.

Beyond food and the microbiome, the intestine has other things to worry about. The sheer number of toxic substances in our homes and gardens makes exposure impossible to avoid. Fertilizers and insecticides can be absorbed directly through the skin. Antifreeze tastes sweet to cats, and licking only a teaspoon of antifreeze that leaks from a parked car is enough to cause kidney failure. But most serious of all is that cats are uniquely vulnerable because they groom themselves with their tongues. Anything that is carried in the air will settle on the cat's fur and be ingested as the cat bathes itself. The list of air pollutants is too long to digest, but cigarette smoke is particularly dangerous. Any cat that lives with a smoker is probably a nicotine addict from licking smoke residue from its fur. Even worse, cats that live with a cigarette smoker have a greatly increased risk of intestinal lymphoma[3]. It would be impossible to eliminate all environmental chemicals, but once a harmful substance is known in the environment it makes sense to minimize the cat's exposure (and our own).

In the cat world, all roads eventually lead back to stress. The digestive tract reacts to environmental changes, lifestyle challenges, and social interactions. We will look at stress and its other health effects more in Chapter 10.

When the cat doesn't feel well inside, life isn't as good as it should be. A large percentage of cats with IBD suffer in silence, but it is hard to know how the cat feels inside because there are few good tests for intestinal inflammation. Exploratory surgery and full-thickness biopsy are the gold standard for diagnosis, but an invasive approach is hardly warranted if symptoms are mild or invisible. One reasonable approach is to be suspicious that any cat that "isn't quite himself", is lethargic, has occasional "hairball vomiting", or passes loose stool is suffering from intestinal disease, and consider treating "as if" a biopsy had shown IBD. The tools that are available for improving intestinal health are similar for most of GI problems:

Try different diets. I usually start with a low-carbohydrate canned food, then move to an easily digestible intestinal diet (often labelled low-residue), then try a higher-fiber diet (or add 1 teaspoon canned pumpkin to the canned food diet), then eventually end up with a true food allergy diet. Each new food will have to be fed for 2 or 3 weeks to judge whether it makes a difference, 8 weeks for the food allergy trial. It is very hard to predict what type of diet will work best, and trial-and-error is needed.

Any time intestinal signs persist for a week or more, a trial on probiotics is warranted. Since we don't know the ideal type of probiotic, some experimentation may be required, rotating different bacterial supplements. One of the only well-controlled studies of probiotics for digestive problems in cats was done by Dr. Lappin at Colorado State University. He used a product by Purina called Fortiflora, and he showed that it reduced the length of diarrhea in cats recently brought to a shelter (the combination of stress and diet change causes diarrhea in most cats) from 3 days to 2 days[4].

If the signs of intestinal upset are moderate to severe, medications may be needed to reduce inflammation so that other treatments can have time to work. The most effective treatment involves some type of cortisone (usually prednisolone). While these drugs carry the risk of side-effects, cats tolerate corticosteroid drugs much better than people or dogs do, and efforts to control IBD without cortisone are usually unsuccessful. Even when prednisolone treatment alone is effective, we try to reduce or eliminate the need for drugs by searching for the right combination of diet and probiotic.

We have come to realize that stress is a common underlying factor for IBD and other intestinal diseases. Drugs, diet, and bacterial supplements may treat improve the bowel symptoms, but the gut is trying to tell us something about the cat's lifestyle. Even occasional vomiting can be a cry for environmental enrichment.

It should be apparent that treating the inflamed intestine is complicated and frustrating. Given how common hidden intestinal problems are in cats, even the healthy cat's digestive system deserves attention. Every cat is different and there is no single approach that will make every cat feel its best, but a reasonable starting point would be simple: feed 1/2 of a 7 1/2oz can of canned kitten food twice a day, along with 1 teaspoon canned pumpkin and a sprinkle of probiotic at each meal. From there, every cat owner is on their own to find the perfect combination for their feline friend.

At the beginning of this chapter we met Ania, my long-haired black cat that periodically vomits hairballs. She has done this periodically for years, but now I know just what to do for her. Many years ago she threw up twice in the same week, and I was curious about whether there might be something going on inside her. I did a brief exploratory surgery (20 minutes from opening to closing) and biopsied her stomach, intestine, liver and a little piece of pancreas. The pathologist reported that Ania's intestine and liver were normal, but she had chronic low-grade pancreatitis. Although her intestine appeared normal, feline pancreatitis has a lot in common with IBD. Because giving a predniso-lone tablet every day seemed like a lot of work (and stress for both of us), I gave Ania a long-acting cortisone injec-tion, and it eliminated the vomiting for 4 months. When she threw up again months later I gave another injection (injectable medication isn't ideal, because if side effects occur the medication is still in the body for a month and we can't take it back) and I switched her to a food allergy diet of venison and pea. After a year or two we gave up on the special diet, since it was hard to tell how much difference it made and other cats in the house made it difficult to feed her separately. Over the past 10 years, Ania has been on a regular premium quality food and is remarkably healthy. She doesn't look like a 19 year-old kitty. Ania has vomiting episodes 2 or 3 times a year, but I know her chronic disease will improve if I give her a small dose of cortisone. We have made feeble efforts to find another diet that agrees with her, but she seems happy with whatever we feed her. When she vomits on the rug I just tell my wife that "she must have a hairball", even though I don't believe it. Ania gets medication any time she throws up twice in the same month—or when my wife steps in a pile of cat vomit when she gets out of bed in the morning.

CHAPTER 9: LET'S BE FRIENDS—OR NOT

A paw reached out through the cage door, pleading "Take me home, please!". My wife and I had gone to the animal shelter looking for a new cat. One of our household kitties had recently passed away and the house seemed somehow lonely, despite my wife and myself, our two children, our Golden Retriever, and two other cats. As the paw reached out again, we looked closer at the cage's occupant. She was still an adolescent, a shorthaired grey tabby with a faint mottling of orange; we have always preferred long-haired cats, but this cat really seemed to be calling out to us. After looking over the other cats we found another gray cat with medium fur and an appealing face that we decided to adopt. But as we walked by the first cat again she meowed plaintively at us. We ended up bringing both cats home and a long and complicated relationship was born.

It seems that the experience of a cat "choosing" a person with whom to live is common, whether it is a bedraggled stray who "just shows up" or the plaintive shelter orphan. Half of the clients who bring their newly adopted kitty to see me report that they formed an immediate connection with their cat, even though they weren't looking for that particular type of pet. None of these new cat owners can tell me what made them decide "this is the pet for me". The feeling is often so intense that it seems tinged with destiny. Adult cats are more likely than kittens to make up their own mind about new people, but perhaps that is only because very young cats are promiscuous in their affections. Older cats have more experience about people to draw upon, but their choices are still a mystery. Just like falling in love, it remains beyond explanation.

Cats have acute senses that must signal something about a stranger immediately and smell may play a part. We each have our own distinct combination of skin chemicals that creates our unique smell and odors have emotional effects that are immediate and powerful. Even more directly linked to the emotions are pheromones, chemicals emitted by the skin and received subconsciously by the cat's vomeronasal organ on the roof of the mouth. I have seen a number of cats that are strongly attracted to people who wear particular pheromone-based perfumes and it may be that our own natural smell has a similar effect.

Smell and pheromones may play a part, but cats are sensitive to other less obvious signals from people. Body language is fluently spoken by cats, and they pick up on subtle cues from our eyes, face, and posture. They may also sense our skin's temperature and electrical charge, but what they think is an attractive sensory signature is opaque to us. Maybe they just know something that we don't.

We named our new shorthaired cat from the shelter Feather, referring to the way that the gray tabby and orange fur blended in a delicate way around her face. The other cat that we took home that day we named Huckleberry, a tribute to Blueberry, the cat that we had just lost. Huckleberry turned out to be the most affectionate of the many cats that have lived in our family, but her story is for another time. Feather turned out to be an emotional enigma.

We should have known that Feather would be different. The shelter personnel told us that, to the best of their knowledge, she had been born in the woods to a feral mother and had not come in contact with people until her litter was rescued at ten weeks old. The age at which socialization occurs is critical in cats. This period of bonding for kittens ends at eight or nine weeks of age. (Dogs are different; even the dog that has never seen a person until four months of age will quickly accept humans as a kindred species and become socially bonded.) Kittens have only two months after birth to form the emotional imprint that allows them to completely accept humans (or children, or dogs). After the age of nine weeks cats can be tamed to tolerate humans, but they never completely trust them or accept them as family. Human contact may be tolerated, but at the expense of a constant stressful vigilance. This became evident with Feather after we took her home. Unlike Huckleberry, who was the same age, Feather spent much of her time hiding and would scamper away when we came into the room. But she was ambivalent, approaching us as if she craved affection and then refusing to be picked up. Even as an adult, Feather would run away if we stood up; if we sat down she would sit at our feet, and when we laid down she would hop up on our chest and start purring. But even then the slightest movement would send her away again. We eventually concluded that she must have been rescued from the woods just after her socialization period had expired, but there was still enough flexibility to allow for some degree of attempted friendship. Feather truly lived between two worlds, that of a wild feline and that of a house cat.

Some observers have maintained that during the socialization process a young kitten comes to believe that it is actually a human being. In some species, this is an accurate analogy. Konrad Lorenz, the father of the animal behavior science of ethology, is famous for describing how geese that he adopted as newly hatched goslings followed him as if he was their mother, and as adults they would ignore their own species and act like Lorenz was their mother, comrade, and potential mate. This is not the sort of identification that cats make when they socialize to humans. Rather, they know that they are part of the cat community, but they willingly join the human community as well, happy to have it both ways, a sort of dual citizenship. In this chapter we will look first at the many and varied relationships that develop between cats and people, and then examine how cats interact with other cats. But being the individuals that they are, any generalization we make about the social life of cats can be contradicted when a cat chooses to define its own relationships.

Once upon a time, not that many years ago, we imagined that cats were a solitary non-social species that maintained separate territories and met up only for procreation. This idea came from our limited imaginations. The human concept of a social relationship was confined to our familiar human interactions. The domestication of dogs reinforced this idea; we could understand their social structure, and the wild canine easily fit into the human family.

During the 20th century the human social sciences came to appreciate diversity in personality, behavior, and culture. In the new millennium animal behaviorists have taken an increasingly open-minded approach to the study of animals, and they have discovered astonishing levels of complexity, even in the "non-social" cat family.

The idea that cats can have personal relationships with humans and other cats rests on several philosophical questions that still generate some controversy. These questions include whether cats possess consciousness, whether they recognize other specific individuals, and whether they have a sense of self.

Philosophers have argued for centuries about whether animals share the quality that we refer to as consciousness. Although people who live closely with animals have always credited cats, dogs, and other domestic animals with a conscious awareness of the world, scientists have largely frowned upon these feelings as anthropomorphic projections. During the past few decades, neuroscientists have used newer forms of imaging (MRI, PET scans, and others) to explore consciousness in humans, and how animals may compare. This discussion is beyond the scope of this book, but we can refer to some of the world's leading neuroscientists in this matter. Cognitive scientists met in 2012 to discuss this very question at the Francis Crick Memorial Symposium on Consciousness at Cambridge University. Dr. Crick was the Nobel Prize-winning co-discoverer of the structure of DNA, and he spent the last part of his career studying how our brains produce consciousness. The world-renowned scientists who met to honor his contributions and carry his work forward ended the historic conference with a two-page statement that was summarized by the statement "Convergent evidence indicates that non-human animals have the neuroanatomical, neurochemical, and neurophysiological substrates of conscious states along with the capacity to exhibit intentional behaviors. Consequently, the weight of evidence indicates that humans are not unique in possessing the neurological substrates that generate consciousness. Nonhuman animals, including all mammals and birds, and many other creatures, including octopuses, also possess these neurological substrates."[1]. We can take it on the best authority of neuroscience that cats are indeed capable of conscious thought.

The development of social relationships depends on the ability to recognize another individual and store memories of how one has been treated by that individual. After all, if we don't remember if someone has treated us nicely or rudely then we won't know how to respond the next time we meet them. I still have cat owners that ask me if their cat will remember them when they return after a week-long vacation, as if the feline brain was incapable of holding onto the memory of someone who is central to their life. The evidence is overwhelming that a cat recognizes people that it likes (and especially those that it dislikes) for years. Many cats will immediately greet an old acquaintance that has been long absent by soliciting some ritual that the two shared in the past. Of course, sometimes the cat will pointedly ignore the old friend, but this doesn't mean that the individual isn't recognized; it seems that cats may have their own rules about how long they treat a person who has been gone with disdain. One of my cats was very consistent about this behavior: Every time we left her alone for a weekend she would completely ignore us for exactly 18 hours after our return, and then she would become overly affectionate, as if to say "I had to punish you for leaving me, but I am really glad you are back!". Relationships can be complicated things.

Communication is vital to any relationship, at least according to human popular psychology. Cats certainly make every effort to communicate with the humans in their lives by means of a variety of channels, but our ability to interpret these signals may confound the kitty who may wonder

"Why don't you get it? I was being perfectly clear!". We don't always speak the same language. Humans like to claim that language, complete with words and grammar, is the pinnacle of communication (although an oft-quoted Stanford University language study claims that words make up only 30% of human communication). Dogs have been shown to be adept at deciphering people's words, but cats appear to have limited comprehension of these units of human speech. Elizabeth Marshall Thomas made an observation that reveals how felines can realize that human words carry information, but still be unable to decode what that information is[A]. When she lived in Africa Ms. Thomas had both a German Shepherd Dog and a tame lion. The dog, the lion, and the woman shared an amicable relationship. When Ms. Thomas took the animals for their evening walk, she would verbally announce whether they would be leaving by the front door or the back door. When the dog heard her it would immediately head for the appropriate door (skeptics might claim that the dog was using non-verbal cues like body language to understand her intent, but Ms. Thomas is an experienced anthropologist and animal behaviorist and I would accept her interpretation of the dog's response). However, if the lion was the only animal in the room when she made the announcement, it seemed to be confused about which door would lead to the walk, apparently being unable to decipher the words. This inability to understand human words is understandable, since dogs have had tens of thousands of years of listening to our language. But the lion was not clueless. When both the dog and the lion were present in the room, the lion would respond to Ms. Thomas' announcement by immediately looking to the dog. By taking a cue from the dog the lion appeared to know immediately which way to go, in many cases heading in the right direction before the dog made any perceptible movement. The conclusion that Ms. Thomas came to was that the dog understood her words, and the lion understood the dog. (As a side note, wolves, even those raised by humans, are also very poor at learning human words; this skill only came with canine domestication).

This observation does not mean that we shouldn't talk to our cats. As the Stanford studies established, tone of voice and body language comprise 70% of human communication, and this percentage is probably closer to 95% in many animals, including cats. Experience tells us that cats can grasp much of our meaning from our tone of voice and body language, although that doesn't guarantee that they will comply with our instructions. When we sternly tell our cat to "Get off of the table!", it is very likely that we will be ignored, not because the cat doesn't understand our meaning, but because it has its own idea about what it wants to do. You can almost imagine the cat giving a non-verbal response of "You're not the boss of me!". Most cat owners will agree that their pet often behaves in a way that deliberately challenges human instructions and rules.

For many years my veterinary clinic was home to a pair of littermates, Roxy and Muffy. We had adopted the pair when they were abandoned kittens, and they thrived on all the attention that they received from my staff. There were rules, however. Our hospital had an upstairs where the staff lounge, doctor's office, and manager's desk were located. Because we feared for these adventurous cats if they roamed the active part of the clinic where a dog might get loose and attack them, our rule was that Roxy and Muffy were allowed to roam anywhere in the upper level of the clinic, including the stairs. They learned this rule in a matter of days from the scoldings that staff members gave them any time they were found downstairs. Within a week Roxy and Muffy almost never ventured from their upstairs sanctuary, and when they occasionally explored the downstairs hallway a quick look and a "Get back upstairs!" was enough to send them scampering back up the stairs; they clearly understood that they were in forbidden territory. But that didn't mean that they would obey the house rules. If one of our staff (particularly myself) was standing within view of the bottom of the stairs, Roxy would often perch on the bottom stair and make eye contact as she stretched out her paw toward the forbidden floor. There was no doubt that she enjoyed teasing us in this way, and when we scolded her she would make an exaggerated dash back up the stairs.

I have heard dozens of accounts from my clients about similar playfully defiant cat behavior. When Princess, a tabby owned by a long-time friend and neighbor, was told to get off the kitchen counter, she would walk over to a glass flower vase and push it close to the edge of the counter. Then she would pause with a look that said "If you take one step closer, the vase is gonna get it!". The intent was unmistakable and the first few times this occurred my friend backed off and let the cat have its way (the behavior was sort of cute, in a "make-my-day" kind of way). Finally my friend called the cat's bluff and moved forward to push the cat from the counter—and Princess made good on her threat, the vase crashing to the kitchen floor.

In this case, the communication was all non-verbal, as is most interaction between people and their cats. They often manage to make their wishes (or demands) known to us in ways that are subtle. But they do have voices, and attentive cat people often tell me that they can understand many variations of their cat's talk. The insistent meow is easily interpreted as "I want something", and once we become close to an individual cat we can distinguish between the "feed me", "let me jump up on your lap", and "I want to go outside" vocalizations. Growls are a universal language, and we are well advised to pay attention. A quiet sound that is usually described as "chuffing" is sometimes used in an intimately friendly interaction, although the sound is subtle enough that it may escape human notice. More obvious and to the point is a peculiar deep whining sound that is most often associated with a successful hunt. Cats that catch mice often seem to announce their success with this sound, usually while carrying their dead prey inside to show off to their owners. Although this sound is almost always used in a "look what I have" context, the object of the cat's bragging can vary. One of my cats would make the noise when it found a sock in the laundry and carried it around the house. Other cat people report their cat's own variations on this theme: a scrap of paper for one cat, a found penny for another. Strangely, I rarely ever hear of cats making this sound when they catch a bird. We can't understand the thoughts behind everything a cat says.

It often seems like cats expect us to understand what they are saying, which is a little surprising, since cats prefer to communicate among themselves with body language and scent. Some cats are very chatty with people, regaling their owners with a constant stream of feline commentary; Siamese cats are particularly famous for their loquacious natures. It is my impression that these cats observe people talking and imitate the activity. When the cat imitates their owner's talkativity, it may do it as a way to join in and be involved with a human activity that it doesn't understand, rather than to communicate some particular intent or desire.

Purring is used by a mother cat to soothe her kittens, but is adapted for other uses, such as expressing contentment and beguiling us into continuing to do what the cat wants. Purring also has other meanings beyond contentment. We frequently hear terminally ill cats begin to purr when they are nearing death. Whether this is due to the euphoric feeling produced by a flood of endorphins during the cat's final hours or something more mysterious is hard to say. It comforts me to think that the cat's passing is not overshadowed by suffering.

Purring is a fascinating mystery in other ways. Purring creates vibrations at a rate of 26Hz (twenty six cycles per second, the frequency of the lowest note on a piano), but the sound is not created by activating the vocal cords, as in other vocalizations[2]. Small laryngeal muscles oscillate in a slightly out-of-phase manner with the diaphragmatic muscles to vibrate the column of air in the windpipe without interrupting airflow in and out of the trachea. The cat can even use the vocal cords to make other sounds without interrupting the purr, in a dual-channel communication system. Researchers have discovered that cats have several types of purr: The basic 26Hz purr is usually associated with relaxation and contentment, while a second "solicitation purr" adds a higher frequency tone to the mix[3]. This two-tone purr carries a message that the cat wants something. Even non-cat owners can tell the difference between these purrs, rating the enhanced purr as "more urgent and less pleasant" than the basic purr.

Purring may serve more complex functions as well. The same 20+Hz frequency of vibration is used therapeutically in humans to speed healing, restore damaged muscle, and dampen pain[4]. Some anecdotes have suggested that fractures and injuries recover more quickly when a purring cat is snuggled up next to the patient, but we don't know whether this is an evolutionary adaptation that the cat can consciously direct to enhance physical recovery for itself and its family, or whether it is just a happy coincidence that the cat's contented communication runs at the same frequency that stimulates cellular healing. Either way, the sound of a cat's purr is comforting.

If they had their preference, most cats would likely prefer to let their body do the talking.

Volumes have been written about feline body language. We won't examine this communication channel in detail here, but simply offer a few observations.

When my three young granddaughters got two new kittens, we tried to teach our girls to listen to what their new cats were saying by watching their tails and ears. When the ears went back, we told them, their kitty was displeased with how tightly they were being hugged and it was time to let the cat loose. When the tip of the tail ticked back and forth and the kitten showed other signs of playfulness, then our girls could tell that the game was all in good fun. But when the tail lashed back and forth furiously, we told them, leave the kitty alone; it may not be angry, but certainly it is overstimulated and ready to make what our five-year-old twins call "bad decisions". The lesson is "Listen to the tail."

The feline body has a rich repertoire of communication gestures, but they always need to be interpreted in light of the individuality and creativity of the cat. We often hear behavior experts tell us exactly what a particular posture or movement means, but different cats may be more or less likely to use any particular body language. At a recent lecture, a feline behaviorist stated that cats are put at ease when we blink our eyes slowly at them. The underlying message here is that "I am so friendly and relaxed that I am a little drowsy". I have personally tried blinking slowly at a number of different cats, and I have never noticed any change in their attitude. Maybe I am not saying it right.

In addition to body language, cats can find actions that speak louder than words. They are at their most creative when it comes to demanding that their owner get out of bed to meet the cat's wants. One of our cats, a long-haired black and white female named Casey, would meow at 4AM to remind us that it was only two hours from feeding time, and we might want to take care of that now. We were able to ignore these verbal commands, but this only led to an escalation of the demands. Casey would leap from the bed onto the screen of the window nearest the bed and hang there until we responded in the way that she wanted. This trick was enough to jolt us awake every time. When my son's cat Apollo spent time with us he took a different approach to the morning wake-up, but equally effective. At first he would knead on my chest with his front paws, a normal kitten nursing behavior that is often used by adult cats to convey affection with just a hint of neediness. When this failed he would give a few little head bumps. If these were ignored he would rest one of his fangs against my cheek, gently at first, and then leaning more of his weight onto the tooth. I don't think that he was threatening to bite, but this tactic was impossible to ignore and the point was made.

No matter how well we try to listen to cats and communicate with them, there is no substitute for the attitude that we bring to every feline encounter. The best way to describe this is spelled R-E-S-P-E-C-T. In my veterinary experience, when cats are treated with respect they are often willing to tolerate things that they naturally find objectionable, such as taking medication. In the veterinary hospital the power of a respectful attitude is magnified. Too often veterinarians have used the farm-animal traditions of forceful restraint, which can be counter-productive when handling cats that are nervous, frightened, or non-compliant. In my own three-doctor practice the veterinarians and technicians were required to handle cats as if we were asking them for their cooperation, rather than forcing them to our wills. When a cat declined to come out of its carrier for an examination, we would dismantle the carrier and examine the cat as it sat in the bottom half of the crate. When something truly objectionable was necessary, a large towel was draped over the cat and folded to allow access the area of interest. And above all, "scruffing" cats was forbidden. It is unfortunately still a common practice in some veterinary clinics and shelters to grasp the cat by the loose skin over the shoulders and lift it for restraint. But cats don't like it and forgiveness is not a feline virtue.

After leaving my own veterinary practice I have worked at dozens of other veterinary hospitals as a temporary "re-lief" veterinarian and I have observed a wide range cat-handling styles. In many veterinary clinics the staff has been trained to scruff cats when handling them; the techni-cians usually tell me that they must handle cats in this way or they would be bitten, since most cats are uncooperative. By the time I have a chance to examine a cat that has been roughly handled, it usually lives up to its bad reputation. But at many other veterinary hospitals the doctors and staff tell me that they never scruff cats and they rarely find them difficult to handle. The cats are the same; the only differ-ence between the clinics where heavy restraint is used and those where cats are cooperative is the respect accorded to the feline patients.

Whether in the veterinary clinic or lounging around the house, cats have strict standards of how they want to be treated: Be respectful, avoid being demanding, approach obliquely, and have a little sense of humor—your kitty may just be teasing you.

Cats live in a world of many different relationships. The associations between people and cats are often overshadowed by the interactions of cat with their own species. As discussed previously, cats are not the non-social loners that we once believed. Their relationships with other cats are complex and often unpredictable.

In multiple cat households, groups of cats often form convivial groups that share sleeping areas, groom each other, and greet one another with obvious affection. Many times group members are related, a female with grown offspring. Males tend to hang out with other males, although this is as variable as every other feline behavior. Sometimes it is a mystery why two cats become friends. We met Feather earlier, our poorly socialized, nearly feral grey and orange female. At the time our house had three other cats, including Puffy, a seal-point Himalayan retired show cat that had come to live with us because her owner could not deal with her urinary behavior problems. Both Feather and Puffy largely ignored the other cats in the house, but they immediately became best friends, sharing grooming sessions and resting with their paws draped over each other. It was difficult to imagine what these two very different cats could have in common: It was as if a girl from the wrong side of the tracks became lifelong friends with a society debutante. As with feline attraction to particular people, they must have reasons for friendship which are hidden from us.

When owners ask me if they should get another cat to keep their single pet company, I usually counsel that they should get another cat only if they want one themselves. From the cat's perspective, an additional cat may be welcomed or rejected; most cats find some middle ground between tolerance and friendship, but it is impossible to predict. There is one exception, however. If two kittens from the same litter are available to be adopted together it is always a positive situation. Not only can the kittens become perfect playmates, but they seem to draw confidence and reassurance from each other. Pairs of littermates are the most well-adjusted and happy cats that I see.

It is easy to understand why cats may develop animosity to other cats. First impressions are important, and often indelible. This is why we recommend keeping a new cat in a separate room for the first week after it joins a new household. If the newcomer is forced to come face to face with a nervous resident cat, there may be hissing and scratching. This can fuel a life-long animosity between these cats that could have been avoided. Even with gradual introductions, cats can develop individual dislikes as easily as they make friends. These rocky relationships fuel many of the problem behaviors and stress-driven health problems of cats. Surprisingly the animosity between household cats can be so subtle that the owners are not even aware of the tension. The most common manifestation of trouble in paradise involves the litter box.

Urine spraying and "inappropriate elimination" are behavior issues routinely seen by veterinarians, and while there are many reasons why a cat will urinate or defecate outside of the litter box, an uneasy relationship with other cats is the most common. "Cat box politics" can be as devious and underhanded as human politics. If a cat owner starts finding evidence of urination in secluded corners of the house (most often on a carpeted floor), we often find that one of the other cats is silently intimidating the cat with "The litter box is mine, stay out" messages. One way that a dominant cat may make its point is by defecating in the litter box and refusing to bury the feces. When owners insist that intimidation has nothing to do with a cat's errant eliminations, we sometimes have them videotape the cats while the owner is gone. The video often reveals that the intimidator simply lays in a strategic spot where the victim has to pass on its way to the latrine. We see the more submissive cat repeatedly approach the spot that the other cat has controlled and then retreat again. You can't blame the cat that is threatened for choosing a safer option and urinating in some unauthorized area.

This description may sound like life in a multi-cat household has all of the drama and danger of a cell-block in a human prison, but in many cases it is more friendly feline competition than real threat of bodily harm, more college dorm than state penitentiary. In any case, feline relationships can often be eased by providing a generous choice of litter pans in different parts of the house, as well as plentiful resting and hiding spots.

Even when true dislike surfaces between cats in the same house, it is extremely rare for household cats to actually inflict harm on each other. This is somewhat surprising, considering how regularly cats are injured by other cats in neighborhood spats. Different rules clearly apply.

Interactions between cats outside of the house fall into a variety of discrete categories: Establishing territory for a new cat, border disputes with established neighbor cats, free-ranging aggression from stray male cats, and even friendly encounters with nearby residents.

Cats can have relationships with outdoor cats with whom they have never been in contact with. Usually this takes the form of outside cats patrolling near the inside cat's home, perhaps making noise and spraying urinary "death threats" around the windows and entrances in the house. The cat that is safely confined inside is acutely aware of the hostile communications of outdoor cats, and this is one of the most common triggers for the inside cat that starts urine marking the house. Although psychotropic medications can decrease the inside cat's anxiety about the rough neighborhood outside, the ultimate solution would be to convince the stray cats to leave the area.

Sometimes even these "long-distance relationships" can be positive. A number of cats that I know recognize when some particular neighbor cat comes by the house, even though they have never had direct interaction. Their meowing and rubbing against surfaces inside and outside the house gives evidence that two cats can have a friendship that is not fulfilled by direct contact. Even to a human observer it is clear that the cats share some sort of friendship. Is it expressed by sound? By smell? By glimpses through a window? Before we mount skepticism that a relationship requires the participants to share the same room, we should consider some human relationships that exist only over the internet.

Human and feline relationships have many similarities. They can be loyal or fickle, ambivalent or passionate, based on convenience or moved by mysterious invisible bonds. Most of all, these connections are vital to quality of life. In the next chapter we will see how these intangible interactions exert their impact on the cat's health.

Chapter 10: PANDORA'S PROBLEM

The door opens and a young woman walks into a large room filled with eight cats. She leans down to scoop up a tortoise-shell female that greets her by rubbing against her legs. "How are you this morning, Jewel?", she coos as the cat climbs up and perches on her shoulder. "Would you like a little breakfast?"

This scene is not the home of a cat-hoarding eccentric, but a part of the cat colony at The Ohio State University. When we hear about cats and research facilities it is easy to imagine rows of cramped cages with cats who are terrified of their handlers, but this is not the case here. One third of the cats in this vivarium at the OSU College of Veterinary Medicine were relinquished by their owners because of frustratingly intractable bladder problems. Cats that repeatedly suffer bladder inflammation and urinate outside of the litter box can wear down even the most patient cat lover. The remaining cats were healthy cats obtained from a commercial source. In total there are four rooms with eight cats in each area, and all of the cats have participated in studies of health and behavior. Their familiar caretakers are mostly veterinary students. Interacting with their feline charges is a welcome distraction from the interminable lectures in pathology and anatomy, and the cats appeared to appreciate the attention.

Life is predictable in the cat colony. Feeding times are strictly observed and the same two caretakers feed and clean the cattery every day. Prescribed play times of at least fifteen minutes twice daily are required. Each cat has four of its own toys. Quiet classical music (the cats appear to prefer Vivaldi) is piped in. Bedding is laundered weekly, with a vanilla-and-lavender fabric softener added. Life is good.

But in 2011 this research facility was the home of a study that profoundly shaped our ideas about the link between feline emotions, lifestyle, and health[1]. For seventy-seven weeks all cats were monitored closely for any "sickness behaviors" such as vomiting, stool abnormalities, bladder problems, skin disease, respiratory ailments (asthma), and appetite variations. During eleven of these weeks some change in the environment or routine took place. What happened during these periods of change has deep implications for understanding cats and their lives.

Overall, these cats had three times as many sickness behaviors during the eleven weeks of change and stress as they did during the other sixty-six weeks. The most common symptoms noticed were vomiting and painful urination. One unexpected finding was that the increase in sickness behaviors was the same among the cats that had been donated because of recurring bladder problems (known to be stress-related) and the healthy cats. Apparently stress plays a big part in feline health issues.

When I first read the summary of this landmark study, I imagined that these kitties were subjected to highly unpleasant stresses, perhaps being sprayed with a stream of water, or being forced to listen to Metallica at high volume. But the details of the paper gave a different picture. During the "stress weeks", unfamiliar caretakers took over the feeding, cleaning, and attention. Feeding hours were delayed by an hour, playtime was decreased, and Vivaldi was no longer played during the after-dinner hour. These hardly seemed like traumatizing events, and yet they were enough to triple the weekly medical symptoms. What was going on here?

The backstory on the Ohio State study goes back decades. Cystitis has long been one of the most frustrating feline problems. The affected cat strains to urinate, the urine becomes bloody, and the cat often chooses to urinate outside the litter box; whether the kitty blames the litter box for the pain and chooses some other area, or whether the urge to urinate is simply so immediate and intense that there isn't time to get to the box is not clear. These are the same symptoms as a bladder infection, so in the past we would often treat these cats with antibiotics. The problem often resolved, but signs would come back frequently and bacterial cultures were always negative. Frustrated, veterinarians started to blame the food: Too much ash (mineral content), too much magnesium, not enough acidity, or insufficient moisture each took its turn as the nutritional villain, and special bladder care diets were prescribed. But still cystitis persisted as a reoccurring problem.

Our view of feline bladder disease started to change when Dr. Tony Buffington at The OSU Veterinary School noticed a similarity with a stress-induced disease in women called Interstitial Cystitis. The symptoms of Interstitial Cystitis are the same as a bladder infection (worse, I have been told), but no infection or other cause can be found. Because of the similarity between the human and feline disease, the term Feline Interstitial Cystitis (FIC) was coined. Unfortunately, having a new name for the syndrome didn't solve the problem of how to spare these cats from frequent bladder pain.

In the last decade, veterinarians have come to accept that stress is the underlying cause for FIC. Now that we understand this, it is easier to see the pattern: Flare-ups of cystitis commonly follow events like moving to a new house, bringing a puppy or a baby home, or the noise of nearby construction. Our first recommendation in these cases is to try to determine what is stressing the cat and avoid it. More recent studies have examined how providing "environmental enrichment" can be used to treat FIC. Chapter 11 will be devoted to ways to positively enrich the cat's home surroundings, improve life, and treat a variety of ills. It is significant that in the Ohio State University study, twenty of the cats had been donated to the experiment because they had a long history of untreatable bladder inflammation. All of these cats had fewer symptoms after they joined the group of cats in the study. It appeared that a structured lifestyle with the same caretakers, regular feeding times, playtime, grooming, and music had a positive effect on even these most stubborn cases of bladder disease.

The story of stress and health goes even deeper. Humans are known to develop mysterious stress-related illnesses that have been lumped under the name of Medically

Unexplained Symptoms (MUS). In this syndrome, no physical cause can be found but the symptoms are real. Previously MUS may have been referred to as "psychosomatic" illness, with the implication that it is "all in the person's head". While it is true that the brain and nervous system are involved, the effects on the body are not imaginary. One of the best known illnesses that falls under the MUS umbrella is Fibromyalgia, a debilitating disease of aches and pains. Many Fibromyalgia sufferers report that the worst part of the problem is that the disease doesn't seem "real" to friends, family, or employers. "If your pain is caused by stress", an unsympathetic boss might say, "then take a few days off and then get a grip on yourself." Righting the ship of a neurohormonal stress system that has gone out of balance is still a goal that is out of reach. One of the lessons of MUS is that the problems are rarely confined to a single body system. This observation prompted researchers to investigate whether cats with bladder disease might have other health problems.

One of the problems in studying something as vague and pervasive as feline sickness behaviors or MUS in humans is that specialists tend to concentrate only on their part of the body. Asthma doctors rarely look outside of the respiratory system to see what else might be going on, and intestinal specialists may not ask the diarrhea patient about their home life. Previously, FIC was considered to be only a urinary problem, placing it under the banner of the urology specialists. As it happens, Dr. Buffington is a nutritional specialist at Ohio State who had spent decades studying feline bladder problems because it was thought to be a food problem. But he followed where the evidence led, even though he was not a urinary specialist, and he uncovered the link between bladder, stress, and brain. Now that it is established that the cat's reaction to its environment plays a large part in FIC, Dr. Buffington has focused on cat behavior. And as we will see, hormonal abnormalities have been discovered that will expand this search into other specialties as well. The term "holistic" has been stretched and abused at times, but FIC is helping us learn how connected the brain and other body systems are. A new label of "scientific integrative medicine" has been coined to encourage the investigation of these connections.

In the cat colony, stress-related problems were not confined to the bladder, although many cats joined the colony because of long-standing bladder symptoms. Vomiting was the most common sickness behavior, but skin disease, breathing problems, and appetite changes joined bladder problems on the list. This prompted an effort by Dr. Buffington and his group to search for ailments affecting other parts of the body. Once the focus was no longer restricted to just the bladder, a variety of other problems were uncovered[2]. Behavioral abnormalities were found, as well as heart problems, hormonal imbalances, and digestive problems. Many of these changes were functional, rather than the fault of the tissues themselves. In other words, vomiting might occur even when stomach biopsies appeared normal, or the skin may be itchy even when no specific cause could be found. This explains why MUS is so frustrating for human sufferers, and why cats can be afflicted by vague problems that are difficult to pin down. There is a common acronym used informally by all veterinarians: The medical record may note that the cat is presented for "ADR", and every vet knows that this means the cat just "Ain't Doin' Right". Sometimes a cause can be found and treated, but other times the cat remains in the ADR category. Terminology does make a difference in medicine; what we call a problem often determines what we do about it. With the realization that Feline Interstitial Cystitis shares a lot with other "sickness behaviors", a new name has been coined for this group of stress-related health and behavior problems: The Pandora Syndrome[3].

Sapphire and Topaz were littermates and they shared everything. Both were black with luxuriant long hair, and the only way I could tell them apart when they came in for routine visits was that Sapphire was a little heavier and wore a blue collar, and Topaz was less confident. Sapphire was always the first to brush up against me for attention, but Topaz would soon feel left out and jump up to the exam table for her share of petting.

Both cats were healthy and life was uneventful until their 8th year, when a routine examination revealed a firm lump over Sapphire's left shoulder. It didn't seem painful and it would not have normally caused alarm, but in 1995 reports had just surfaced of sarcomas (a type of soft tissue cancer) being found near sites where vaccinations had been given. This was a devastating finding; vaccination had controlled most of the fatal infections of the 1960's (Distemper), 1970's (Rhinotracheitis), and 1980's (Feline Leukemia Virus), but the last thing we wanted to do was to be responsible for causing malignant tumors. We know now that Vaccine-Site Sarcomas are caused by a tumor-causing gene carried by certain cats which is activated by inflammation. Older vaccines were designed to create mild inflammation in order to push the immune system into creating greater immunity to the vaccine virus. Anything that causes inflammation (other injections, injury, cat bites) could trigger the tumor gene, but booster vaccinations were most commonly incriminated. Initially tumors occurred in approximately one out of every ten thousand vaccinated cats. Sapphire was the only cat I ever vaccinated that developed a sarcoma, but I have never gotten over the experience. (Newer vaccines are designed to cause less inflammation and this problem has become even more rare). Sapphire had several surgeries to remove the aggressive tumor over the course of the next year, but eventually had to be euthanized because of the spread of the cancer.

Sapphire's sister Topaz was visibly affected. Cat owners often ask me if cats grieve for their lost housemates; it is obvious from their behavior that cats can suffer emotionally when a dog, cat, or person dies. How they understand death is an open question, but philosophers and theologians have not provided mortal explanations that humans can universally accept, so we can hardly expect more of cats. Suffice it to say that cats develop strong emotional bonds, and when these bonds are torn apart there can be stress and loneliness.

I examined Topaz several weeks later, as she didn't seem to be bouncing back from the loss of her sister. Her appetite was poor, and she seemed to breathe with more effort. It is easy to become a little paranoid when one of our cats dies, and it is natural to wonder if our other cat might also harbor some serious hidden disease. I have seen many cases in which a cat's depression is initially attributed to grief, only to find that there really is a serious but unrelated health problem. To be on the safe side we ran a few tests on Topaz and found no clues. The vague signs persisted for more than a month after Sapphire's death, but Topaz gradually resumed her normal activity and appetite. We could say that these sickness behaviors were just psychological manifestations of grief, but in the context of the Pandora Syndrome it is likely that there was some real physical illness that had been caused by the stress of Topaz' loss. As I look over her old medical records, I suspect that we would have found some heart malfunction if we had done an echocardiogram. Thankfully Topaz recovered and lived an additional decade after this life-changing episode.

When emotions cross paths with physical illness, a deeper investigation into the neurohormonal mechanism is needed. If we measure how the body responds to stress, we might understand why some cats develop sickness behaviors with the slightest provocation, and others seem more resilient. The most logical place to look is the body's chemical response to stress..

To review the most simplified model, the body responds to emotional stress first with an instant burst of adrenaline (also called epinephrine) and its sister norepinephrine (also called noradrenaline, which is found primarily in the brain). These hormones create the familiar feelings of excitement: A racing heart, dilated pupils, increased blood pressure and blood sugar, and sweating (cats only have sweat glands in the pads of their paws, but I can easily guess a cat's emotional stress when I notice sweaty paw prints on my exam table). The adrenaline rush is followed quickly by a flood of cortisone from the adrenal glands. Cortisone has many of the same effects, but they are less intense and last longer. Both hormones function to ready the body for action when some sudden emergency occurs that requires fighting or fleeing.

Since symptoms of Feline Interstitial Cystitis and the Pandora Syndrome are associated with stress, it seems reasonable that the cats who are most susceptible to stress-induced sickness behaviors would show abnormally high levels of both stress hormones. As often happens in science, the unexpected result often sheds the most light. When researchers studied cats with FIC, they found that they produced less cortisol than normal cats and their adrenal glands were significantly smaller[4,5]. These cats were borderline cortisol-deficient. A certain amount of cortisol is secreted even when life is good and the world is calm, and too little of the hormone can cause intestinal discomfort and malaise. At low doses, cortisol is one of the body's "feel-good" hormones, producing a feeling of wellness and euphoria. When cortisol surges it also turns down the production of adrenaline. Essentially the cortisone surge tells the adrenaline-producing cells "I've got this, you can settle down now". Without an appropriate cortisol response, adrenaline production continues unabated and creates the harmful effects of adrenaline excess. The heart and blood pressure are overstimulated and the brain is anxiously overactive. It appears from recent studies that the cats that develop stress illnesses and behaviors have adrenal glands that are unable to produce enough cortisone to handle everyday stress and rein in excess adrenalin production. Perhaps this explains why so many vague feline illnesses respond to a synthetic cortisone like prednisolone; the steroid drug may be making up for the cat's deficient cortisol production.

Stress can often be tracked back through the family tree. In a variety of species (including man), it has been shown that a mother's stress, even before she is pregnant, can change the development of her offspring's stress response[6]. One can easily imagine that a stray female cat who is living on the edge, avoiding feral tomcats, raccoons, and coyotes while searching for adequate food would be stressed enough that her litter of kittens could start life with adrenal glands that are not able to respond to future challenges. When these kittens are rescued and adopted they may be healthy, and as long as their lifestyle provides security and stability they may live the good life. When the cat matures and has to deal with changing homes, boarding in a kennel for a week, the threat of an outside cat that leaves urine-marks around the front door, or the death of a housemate, things come unhinged.

One of the conclusions of the Ohio State University study was that the cats who developed sickness behaviors could remain well if their environment was enriched. Twenty of the cats had been surrendered to the program because they had severe Interstitial Cystitis problems, and even these cats thrived in the environment provided in the cat colony—as long as nothing changed! Our understanding of how to keep cats healthy and happy has been transformed by this new knowledge. The most important factor in the good life for cats is the environment in which they live, and in the next chapter we will make an attempt to describe how we can provide environmental enrichment for cats of differing personalities.

Chapter 11: TO THE GOOD LIFE

Once a magnificent sleek and muscled predator, a flabby male African lion paces back and forth glumly across his small concrete enclosure. He seems oblivious to the sounds of the small crowd of zoo-goers gathered in front of his cage as he circles his tiny space; if a large predator can have a blank look, this would be it. He turns at exactly the same spot, swinging his maned head from side to side rhythmically as he retraces his steps over and over. His coat is patchy and unkempt, and his massive front legs sag at the carpal joints. It is hard to recognize this animal as the legendary monarch of the African savannah.

Not too many years ago, this sad spectacle was typical of large cats exhibited in zoos around the world. This pacing behavior is called stereotypy, a form of obsessive-compulsive disorder. The rhythmic head movements are reminiscent of the swaying seen in autistic children, and the vacant expression is an unmistakable indication that this lion has tuned the world out, retreating into a trance-like state to block out the world. Some people have even suggested that the head movement creates a sort of hypnosis as the cage bars flicker across the cat's visual field.

Biologists, veterinarians, and behaviorists who advocate for the welfare of animals in zoos have recognized the inhumane inadequacy of the old zoo model in which the priority was to give city-dwellers a chance to see wild animals up close. These experts have tried to find creative ways to make life better for confined animals; whether this is even possible is up for debate, but since life in their native habitat is blighted by poaching, harassment, and starvation, returning to the wild is often not even possible. We can make life better for these animals by searching for ways to meet their needs, no matter where they live. Zookeepers were the first to become interested in what we now call "environmental enrichment".

The first (and often most difficult to obtain) need for the no-longer-wild animal is a space to roam that carries at least a superficial similarity to their natural habitat. Since the home range of a wild lion may run across hundreds of square miles of grassland, zoos are hard-pressed to provide the large expanses that allow large cats to roam, hide, and survey their surroundings. But forward-thinking zoos have tried to create larger outdoor environments with logs, tall grass, and small hills that provide areas out of the sight of visiting humans. People may have to strain to get a glimpse of the lion that lies with its mates behind a bushy rise fifty yards away, but the benefit to the lion's nervous system is significant.

Hunting is more than a hobby for wild members of the cat family; nature has provided predators with the drive to chase and capture prey. We can assume that there is no better feeling than sprinting after a fleeing animal and successfully capturing it. Housecats that hunt mice often appear to be disappointed when their catch goes limp, batting the rodent around as if to prolong the thrill of the chase. Zoos are understandably reluctant to stock their lion exhibits with live antelope to satisfy the need to chase and kill, but they find other ways to make the big cats work for their food. Fish may be frozen into tubes of ice that require work by the lion's jaws or meat might be hidden in unpredictable areas so that searching is required.

Lions are more obviously social than most other members of their family, so carefully chosen social groups are created for captive lions. There is risk involved, since lions are notoriously aggressive to anyone they consider an outsider; in the wild, 60% of lion deaths are caused by other lions. But loneliness can be even more detrimental to health and behavior, and with well-planned introductions lions can be kept in pride-like groups.

Almost anything new and interesting can become a plaything, and zoo visitors may notice decidedly unnatural objects such as large rubber balls in the fake African environment of the zoo lion. Investigating new objects seems to be a rewarding pastime for all cats.

Environmental enrichment has improved the welfare of captive lions, leopards, and tigers, and the benefits are visible even to the casual zoo observer. Muscles can be seen under the animals' full and shiny coats. Most importantly, the large cats stop pacing and start to show behaviors that might be seen in their natural environments. We know that the animals are healthier, and we can assume that they are happier as well.

With the success of environmental enrichment for zoo animals, veterinarians and behaviorists have finally started to look at the lifestyles of our pets through the same lens. Cats may have become domesticated (although not completely, many would hold), but they still carry many of the needs of their not-so-distant ancestors and cousins. The working definition of environmental enrichment is to "increase the biologic relevance of the animal's environment". In other words, life is better when it aligns with the lifestyle for which evolution has adapted the animal. We need to envision the lion that hides inside our pampered Persian if we are to improve its health and quality of life.

Scientists like to divide things into categories, and they have proposed a feline version of Maslow's Pyramid of Needs. The American Associate of Feline Practitioners has codified these needs into five "pillars" of cat wellness[1,2,.] Other humane groups have modified these guidelines, and the essence of these lists can be summarized:

1. Space that is ample and safe
2. Nutritionally adequate and interesting food
3. Bountiful resources, including food, water, litter boxes, scratching posts, more litter boxes, and spots for resting and watching
4. Social interaction
5. Ability to express normal behaviors

The addition of one more element of enrichment completes my own list:

6. A pleasing sensory ambience

This chapter is devoted to exploring environmental enrichment for cats. These suggestions are by no means exclusive; cats all have their own personalities and preferences, and perceptive owners may find many other ways of enhancing the quality of life for their cats. The general principles to follow include meeting the cat's evolutionary needs, maintaining good physical health, and decreasing unnecessary stress. It is important to realize that cats hide their emotional stress, so the claim that "My cat looks perfectly content" is irrelevant. We need to appreciate the "otherness" of cats if we are to discover better ways of caring for them.

Just as in the wild, home starts with a space that the cat can call its own. In one study[3], feral male cats wandered over areas up to thirteen hundred acres, while females typically maintained territories one tenth of the males. A rural farm cat may enjoy roaming over forty acres, while the suburban outside cat patrols a yard of a quarter acre or less (although owned cats in the study actually averaged 4.9 acres each, spending more time in their neighbors' yards than their owners realized). Inside cats may live within the confines of a spacious house or a one-room apartment. Within these spaces, some areas will be more relevant to the cat and more frequented, so the actual measurement of the cat's home territory is less critical than the locations of the resources available. Above all the cat wants choices and the ability to separate itself from other residents of the living space when it wants to.

Although it may seem reasonable to provide food, water, and a litter pan in a designated "kitty room", cats often prefer to have these resources separated. Several food dishes may be placed in different rooms, with water dishes in other areas of the house, and all of these distant from the litter box(s). Some cat owners may balk at have having cat stuff in every room of their house, but with ingenuity these can be blended with the decor (OK, maybe not the litter box, but you get the idea). The dry kibble bowl may be hidden in a space behind the couch, while the plate for a morning and evening offering of canned food might find a corner in the kitchen (since most cats will eat their moist food within thirty minutes of offering, it is convenient to pick up the dish after they eat and add it to the pile of dirty dishes in the sink). Water might be provided in a crystal bowl on the bathroom counter; visitors will think the bowl is merely decorative, and only you and your cat will know otherwise. Even the necessary perching places can be blended with the room; a slanted ladder with wide carpeted steps spaced every fourteen inches can double as a useful step stool near a tall bookcase or by the pantry shelves. Choosing the arrangement of furniture in a room can be made more cat-friendly by placing the couch with its back to a large living room window to create a room with a view.

Providing several safe cat retreats is critical to feline peace and calm. Cats can be ingenious about finding their own hiding areas in the house; more than a few times I have been concerned because I haven't seen one of my cats all day and I would go looking for it, wondering if it had gotten outside or was locked in a closet by accident. I would search every possible secluded space without success. An hour later the cat would wander out from some secret place, stretching and yawning contentedly, and I still wouldn't know where the cat had been. Kitty magic, I tell myself.

We can create these spaces for the cat. A cardboard box laid on its side with a blanket in it will suffice. A cat carrier of sufficient size can be adapted to make a comfortable safe space by taking the door off and lining the plastic carrier with a blanket or a piece of clothing that smells like the cat's favorite human. I suggest that the carrier that is used for a safe space at home is not the one that totes the pet to the vet, however.

Privacy is an important resource for the indoor cat, but just as vital is a good perching place, a spot where the cat can view both the frequented rooms in the house and the action outside the house through the windows. Cats seem to feel more control over their environment when they can keep track of the cats, dogs, and people in the neighborhood. In addition there are wonderful birds, bugs, and other small edible creatures that can be observed, if not savored; this may be like the person who enjoys reading a cooking magazine and drooling over the pictures of luscious desserts that they will never enjoy.

An additional feature of a quality perching spot is elevation. Altitude improves the attitude, they say. Most felines will find some favorite spot on top of a dresser or the back of a stuffed chair, but their preference would be to be above human eye level. In the cat shelter in London that we visited in Chapter 7, a long shelf was provided along one wall a half a foot above the head level of the caretakers. All of the feral cats, who could never feel entirely secure and comfortable with humans, could be found on this high spot, contentedly curled up with each other, high and safe. Wherever a kitty loft is situated, adequate space for a full-length stretch is appreciated.

A house is not a home if it isn't secure. If the inside cat feels threatened by cats that it sees and smells in the outside environment, then taking measures to discourage intruders in the yard can be a positive step to take.

Many of these suggestions can be applied to the single inside cat, but the cat's needs are multiplied as more cats are added to the household. The importance of having more food dishes, water bowls, and litter pans in different areas cannot be underestimated. I have had clients who housed ten cats in a nine hundred square foot house with little conflict and no stress-induced health problems; in these cases, however, the cat owner was always careful to provide an abundance of resources, strategically located to allow all the cats ample choices.

Cats care a lot about food. Nutritional adequacy doesn't quite capture the role that eating plays in the cat's quality of life, however. We previously discussed how dry commercial cat foods have been designed to be adequate, convenient, and economical. But "adequate" does not mean "optimal", and current thinking says that we can do better nutritionally. Low-carbohydrate canned food may have nutritional advantages for many cats. But food is more than nutrition for the body, as any person will testify. Food is flavor, fun, and activity. Consider any recent visit to a restaurant: The ambiance, smells, presentation of the food, and taste make dining out a delightful experience. The cat may not get to experience the pleasure of an epicurean night on the town, but we can enhance the total eating experience for our pets.

The hunting process is as entertaining to a cat as perusing the menu at Chez Pierre might be to us. It would be nice if the cat's food would make an attempt to escape, allowing the cat to pounce on it and subdue each feisty piece of kibble. No one has invented an ambulatory cat food, but there are a variety of food puzzles and cubes that challenge the cat by dispensing a few pieces of dry food at a time when the cat manipulates the feeder in some way. Working for a meal enhances the experience of eating. Many cat owners create the foraging experience by hiding a half-dozen food treats at different locations around the house before they leave for work. Once the cat understands that a little hide-and-seek will reveal a goodie, it will look forward to the game. Even feeding the regular meals in small amounts in different locations can break the routine of eating.

Much of the research on using food as an antidote for stress has found that canned food is helpful in controlling cystitis and other stress-driven diseases. Part of this effect may be the lack of carbohydrates in these foods, but it appears that there is a role for what is called "hedonics"—the sensations involved with eating. Smell may play even more of a role for cats in the enjoyment of food than it does for humans. For sick cats we will often heat canned cat food in the microwave for fifteen seconds and stir it around to release enticing odors to stimulate the appetite. Along with taste, the feeling and texture of food in the mouth completes the sensory experience of a pleasurable meal. This often comes into play with canned food preferences; some cats love "chunks in gravy" foods, while others prefer a blended paté consistency. None of these things can completely recreate the feeling of eating a fresh-caught mouse: the chase and capture, the feel of the cat's fangs popping through the membranes of the mouse's skin, the blending of the tastes of different organs. But that isn't something that most cat people would choose to witness at feeding time. Let's settle for a tablespoon of chunky canned food offered in two different locations, and a handful of kitty treats hidden for later discovery.

The dining experience isn't the only feline activity that involves hedonics. Much human frustration surrounds the litter pan. As convenient as it is for the indoor cat to eliminate in a designated toilet area, it is here that the relationship with our cat often breaks down. What the cat owner wants is for the cat to unfailingly eliminate in the litter box, for odor to be absent, and for minimal time to be required to keep the elimination area clean. What the cat wants is the ability to eliminate undisturbed in a secluded, spacious, and secure location where it is comfortable to enter and leave the box, with a litter substrate that feels good on the paws and has no objectionable odor. These human and feline desires are not always compatible. If these wishes conflict, some cats will eliminate in unacceptable areas (the most common "behavior problem" that is presented to veterinarians). Other cats grudgingly use the inadequate toilet situation, but it adds one more household stress.

To a cat, the elimination area is special real estate, and it follows the axiom of "location, location, location". Especially in multiple cat households, there is a lot of hidden competition, silent aggression, and stress associated with the litter box. The first rule that any cat behaviorist will cite is that the number of litter boxes should equal the number of cats, plus one. They should be in different locations. In many houses a single litter pan can serve several cats, but any time elimination occurs outside of the provided space (or any two cats don't seem to be getting along), more locations need to be added. Since privacy is desirable for this function, the areas less frequented (by both humans and particularly the other cats) are usually chosen. However, cats seem to feel that they are vulnerable while urinating and defecating, so the location should have an easy "escape route" in case of unwelcome interruptions. For this reason, the back of a closet or a narrow alcove with a limited entrance are poor choices. This need for a fast getaway also makes covered cat boxes undesirable. As anyone who was bullied by larger kids in elementary school can relate, you really don't want to be trapped in a toilet stall when the mean kids come looking for you.

Size matters as well. Usually bigger is better, although some older cats may find it painful to step up over the edge of a high-sided cat pan, and they may make bad choices when it hurts to step into the litter pan. Many geriatric cats will put their front legs in the box, leaving their rear legs outside, defeating the purpose of the box. Lower sides may help keep the whole cat in the litter box, and when this doesn't work we can place the litter box on a soft disposable pad (a puppy training "pee pad") extending out six inches around the box to absorb anything that doesn't make it to the litter.

Once we have enough boxes in the right locations, it's what's inside that counts. Pet suppliers provide a dizzying array of materials to soak up urine: Clay, sand, recycled newspaper, walnut shells, plastic beads, and just about anything else that can be ground up for cats to pee on. The list of additives is even longer: baking soda, deodorants, and more synthetic scents than a perfume store. Which one is best? The answer is: Whatever the cat wants. Studies show that the average housecat is most likely to prefer a fine, sandy, clumping litter. Even more important is that the litter is odorless; a scent that reminds humans of a field of flowers is overwhelmingly intense to kitty nostrils, and the cat is likely to express its disapproval by selecting another place to eliminate. Once more, every cat is an individual and entitled to its own preferences. In some cases we will offer a smorgasbord of six boxes lined up side by side with six different litters, letting the cat expresses its own wishes. If a little olfactory enhancement is desired, a small scoop of fresh garden dirt can add an outdoorsy scent to your cat's favorite clumping litter. The important thing about providing a pleasurable elimination experience is to cater to your cat's whims. What kitty wants, kitty gets.

What is a home without a family? Social interactions are basic to quality of life, but there are so many relationship combinations to consider that the best we can do is to be sensitive to the cat's likes and dislikes with other cats, people, and dogs. Clients often feel guilty about leaving their cat alone at home all day, and they ask if they should adopt another cat as a friend. While there is no doubt that feline friendships can be beneficial, there is no way to predict whether a second cat will be a comforting companion or an aggressive annoyance. One of the most clear-cut cases of stress cystitis occurred in my household when my sister-in-law moved to an apartment where she could not keep Miranda, her dark sealpoint Siamese. One of the occupational hazards of being a veterinarian is serving as an orphanage and halfway house for friends and family who need a place for their pet to stay for a while. Miranda came to live with us at five years of age, at a time when we already had five cats in our house. This new addition got along with four of our cats, but she just didn't like Snowy, the old gentleman of the house.

Miranda and Snowy never fought or even hissed at each other, but they glared with displeasure every time they passed in the hallway. Miranda developed Feline Interstitial Cystitis, but this was years ago, before we understood the stress connection. Whenever Miranda would show blood in her urine or strain in the litter box, we would put her on whatever the current medication was for the condition. But like many other cat owners, I could not get her to take a pill at home, no matter how hard I fought with her. Since I was able to give her medication with the help of my staff at the clinic, I would take her to the hospital to stay during her five days of treatment, and each time she would improve rapidly. The third time she had an attack of cystitis I had a revelation; perhaps she didn't get better because of the medication, but simply because she had a vacation away from our house—and Snowy. The next time I kept Miranda at the clinic for five days, but without medication, and she improved just as quickly. Unfortunately, she still had to come home to our house, but now we knew that she just needed a few days of rest and relaxation at the "spa" to get away from it all. After several years of this, my sister-in-law finally moved to an apartment where she could once again keep Miranda, and her cat never had another episode of cystitis. It was years later that Dr. Buffington discovered what I had learned with Miranda: being pissed off can cause peeing problems.

Most feline relationships could be described as ambivalent; sometimes it is nice to curl up with a friend and share a grooming session, but in many instances cats merely tolerate their feline housemates, and sometimes having a companion is a constant irritation. The decision to add another cat to the household is usually made because of the owner's desires, or for the welfare of a cat in need of a home. Gradual introductions are important, and it is advisable to isolate a feline newcomer in its own room for the first week to avoid any unpleasant confrontations. In most cases, with a little sensitivity and an abundance resources spread throughout the house, cats will build a network of relationships with other cats that works for them. But sometimes the only road to domestic tranquility is to find a different place for one of the cats to live.

Cat owners often worry about how their new cat will get along with the family dog, but they usually have nothing to worry about. When Fido comes face-to-face with the new cat, he will usually get the full feline treatment: hissing, arched back, and maybe even a sudden cat-slap in the face (with retracted claws). This is enough to convince the dog to be respectful to the new guest, and once the dog under-stands who is boss the cat will usually be magnanimous enough to tolerate, or even cuddle up to, the dog. Occa-sionally I do see a cat that is stressed by a rambunctious puppy who ignores the cats' refusal to tolerate rough-and-tumble play, but this usually resolves within a week or two.

People matter a lot to cats, even though we may feel like mere servants. In the Ohio State study, the cats were hap-piest when they were always cleaned and fed by the same pair of caretakers. The weeks when a stranger took over the feeding, cleaning, and petting were the times when stress-induced sickness behaviors increased. Sometimes it is hard to discern why cats prefer certain people, but once these bonds are formed they are durable. A positive relationship with a person may be formed by meeting the basic needs and filling the food dish on command, but in many cases the owner who takes care of the feeding and cleaning is disappointed when their pet prefers some other family member. When food fails, there is always touch. Petting is the human equivalent of the grooming that maintains relationships between cats, and physical affection can be a potent enrichment for the cat's life. Although it is natural for us to stroke the top of the cat's head, that may not be what the cat would choose. The most desirable "sweet spot" for petting is under the chin and along the cheeks, avoiding the sensitive whiskers. The "friendly pheromones" produced by skin glands on the side of the face can create an immediate bond when petting the cheek scents the person's fingers. It seems that cats make their judgements about people based on things that are intangible, or at least invisible to us. Smell almost certainly has something to do with this, whether it is a person's individual smell or the scent of a shampoo or cologne that they use. There are times when a person (often the new spouse of the cat's significant someone) is greeted with indifference or outright disdain, despite their best efforts to make friends. The best a person can do is to avoid trying too hard, playing hard-to-get by ignoring the cat until it feels compelled to make its own advances. And sometimes we have to accept that the cat just isn't that into us.

An important part of environmental enrichment might be termed "occupational therapy". For cats as well as humans, mood and well-being are improved by having something to do. Ideally this involves a mixture of predictable routine activities (riding the bus to work for the human, jumping up on the bathroom sink for a drink from the faucet for the cat) and novel adventures (a day on the ski slope for the person, a leash walk at the park for the cat).

Allowing, and even encouraging, normal cat behavior can is important. When we think about inviting the expression of cat behaviors, we have to consider cats in their natural environment: They want to explore, so a new object like a large empty paper bag will attract their attention. They want to play and pounce, making toys that appeal to their predatory instincts irresistible. They want to watch their environment, so a perch with a view satisfies their need to watch and climb.

Scratching household objects may be the least welcome normal feline activity, but a clearer understanding of the cat's motivations can help establish a cease-fire in the conflict between the cat and the couch. In the wild cat's environment, there is usually a single upright object in the most prominent area of cat's territory. The cat uses this to advertise its possession of the area, along with some personal information. Stretching to its full height, the cat will start a long continuous groove down the length of the chosen object to provide a visual sign of how large the territorial owner is (if they could, they might even stand on a stepladder to exaggerate their mighty proportions). Chemicals from the pads of the cat's paws anoint the post with the cat's scent to leave no doubt as to who lives there. None of this has much to do with sharpening claws.

When we provide a scratching post for our cat, we usually get everything wrong, and then wonder why the cat still prefers to maul good furniture. First, the cat has the urge to scratch a vertical object that is central to its home, obvious to all newcomers. Why would we hide the scratching post in some back room of the house? Who wants to advertise to an empty space? Second, many commercial scratching posts are only two feet high, hardly enough height to make a statement about how big the cat is. Third, and perhaps most importantly, cats prefer a material with a long "drag", so that the claw marks can start as high as possible and continue uninterrupted all the way down the post.

Most available scratching posts are covered with carpet, which is sure to catch the claws and destroy the rewarding feeling of the claws skidding along the surface. This explains why the cat's favorite scratching target is often a chair covered with a smooth fabric (for the feeling of the continuous drag of the claws) that is located at the opening to the living room (what more obvious place to advertise to newcomers?).

This what my cats tell me they want for a scratching post: Take a commercial scratching post, at least thirty-six inches tall. Re-cover the post with a fabric like corduroy, with the grooves of the material running in a vertical direction; a staple gun and one yard of fabric should accomplish this quickly. Position the new scratching post in a prominent area where people enter the living area of the house. (Note: once the cat establishes this post as its preferred scratching object, you may be able to move it gradually to a less obvious location). Run your own hands and fingernails up and down the fabric-covered post (admit it, is feels kind of good, doesn't it?). Now the simple scratching post becomes an outlet for normal, pleasurable feline behavior. And you might also keep your kitty's claws clipped, just in case.

When stress happens, some people deal with it by heading for the spa, where the senses are caressed and cared for. Soft music, selected aromatherapies, and dim lights have charms to sooth the savaged nervous system. Feline senses are famously more sensitive than our own, and we underestimate how the wrong smell or sound can get on their nerves. Since many of the aspects of the cat's environment are outside of the range of our sensations, we may not have a clue to what is affecting our cats.

Of the cat's super-senses, smell likely has the strongest effects on health and happiness. We have discussed how a slight whiff of urine marking from a stray tom cat can cause anxiety and distress, but it is harder to judge the positive or negative effects of the normal household smells. Many cleaning agents, including fabric softeners, bathroom cleaners, and good old chlorine bleach are more offensive to the feline nose, creating stress rather than relieving it. Humans seem to like strong-smelling household products; one story tells how the household odor eliminating spray Febreze initially failed to sell. It did a great job of destroying household odors, but it left—no smell! Consumers weren't satisfied just because they could no longer sniff the sweaty laundry and last night's fish dinner; they wanted a smell that told them that the bad odors were gone. A "clean" smell was added to the product, and it was a hit. We don't know how the cats feel about the artificially "fresh" odor of deodorizers, or about the smells of our dish soap, underarm deodorant, or the poly-fill in our couch and pillows. On the other hand, we do know of some pleasant scents that qualify as enriching for cats. Musk-based colognes in tiny doses appeal to many cats with a reminder of their true wild nature. Peppermint, used sparingly (remember, we don't even need to be able to smell it ourselves) shares the attraction of catnip, another enjoyment for many cats. Some novel smells seem to appeal to the exploratory tendencies of many cats: allspice and almond extract are only a few interesting options. And then there are the aromatherapy products that advertise their abilities to calm the human emotions. Some would argue that the power of suggestion plays a dominant role in people's reaction to customized smell therapy, but there have been good studies using lavender aromatherapy to confirm its positive power over feline stress.

Beyond the world of conscious smells are the pheromones, chemicals produced by the body to directly affect the emotions. The cat rubs its cheek against familiar friends and places to mark them with a feeling of calmness, goodwill, and ownership, improving its surroundings in the same way we might hang our favorite family photograph to make a place feel familiar and homey. A synthetic version of the facial pheromone is available as a spray or a plug-in diffusor to help anxious cats get through stressful times or feel more at home.

The household soundscape also deserves attention. Many of the cats that I treat with anxiety or stress diseases seem to be sensitive to noises that we take for granted: Traffic on the nearby highway, a construction project down the street, or surround-sound television and music blaring at volumes that even humans were never intended to endure. We should remember that cats are able to hear even the underground chatter of rodents in their burrows from a distance—a critical skill for the professional hunter, but a liability when the housecat now lives in a small house with a teen-aged drummer, a dishwasher, a clothes dryer, and the weekend activity of power tools in the garage. These sounds are so baked into our modern life that it would be difficult to significantly bring down the noise, but our cats would appreciate the effort. There are unheard sounds as well; humming of the small parts in our electronic gadgetry that are above the range of our hearing, closer to the frequency range of the chatter of rodents in their burrows.

But not all sound is noise to the cat's ears. Certain sounds may be soothing, and low levels of pleasant sounds may help block out unpleasant noises. There has been recent interest in how animals perceive and appreciate music, and whether they can identify with the rhythmic patterns and melodic motifs of human music. Some of the ideas about calming music for cats come from the wishful-thinking school of music, but it does seem to be true that classical music enriches the cat's environment (as well as our own). It may be that cats find orchestral music particularly fetching, since violins and flutes share the frequencies of mice and bird vocalizations. In the Ohio State study, the cats enjoyed Vivaldi's music every day, and this melodic flowing music was one of the factors that provided environmental enrichment and decreased the number of symptoms that the cats suffered. In my own veterinary hospital, and at other clinics where I have consulted, a carefully selected soundscape of classical music or New Age sounds were used in the areas where cats were kept. Did it help the cats? I am not sure, but at least it prevented the kennel help from blasting something less enjoyable as they worked.

Looking over this long litany of feline enrichment, many of these factors bring to mind life in the outdoors, which raises a thorny controversy: Should cats be allowed outdoors? Life outside the house is certainly richer in sights, varied sounds, and smells. Normal cat behaviors, such as digging into soft dirt, scratching trees, and patrolling a defined territory, come naturally for the outdoor cat. Even eating mice and birds can be a healthy addition to the diet, just as the activity of the hunt brings enjoyment. The outdoor lifestyle is inherently healthier than being confined to a house with stale air, unnatural sounds, and other annoying cats and people that can't be avoided. Outdoor cats have less dental problems, less heart problems, and less bladder disease by a factor of ten. And yet cats in this country are increasingly kept indoors. What is the matter with allowing your cat access to the great outdoors?

For one thing, life is dangerous out there. Cat fights are a fact of life, and although an infected bite wound is serious until it is treated, it would be very rare for a cat bite abscess to become fatal, with the exception of the deadly viruses (Feline Leukemia Virus and Feline Immunodeficiency Virus) that may be carried by the bad boys who inflict the bites. Cars, coyotes, poisons, and the infectious diseases carried by stray cats do present a clear and present danger to be considered. In one older study, the lifespans and diseases of inside cats and outside cats were compared. The diseases of each group were predictably different, but the lifespan differential was eye-opening: The inside cats averaged a 15 year lifespan, while the outdoor cats lived an average of only three years. And yet, many very humane-oriented veterinarians, like behavioral specialist Dr. Nicholas Dodman from Tufts University[F], have suggested that, despite the risks, it is kinder to allow cats access to the world outside of the house. Sometimes cats just need to be cats.

A different argument is made by urban/suburban wildlife advocates. Hunting is a normal cat behavior, and one that brought our species together in partnership. But cats are too skilled at it. Cats have been blamed for plummeting populations of songbirds, and our pets have been reviled by bird lovers across the world. This issue has become a standoff, cat lovers against bird lovers, and there seems no easy resolution.

Observations from my own veterinary experience suggest some reasonable middle ground: Allow your cat outdoors only during daylight hours and limit outdoor freedom when your cat is young. For the adult cat, bad things usually happen at night. Automobile injuries are reduced when motorists can see the cat that streaks across the road, and ninety percent of cat bite wounds can be avoided by limiting outdoor activity to daylight hours. Many of the other hazards of outdoor life occur predominantly in young cats. Cats, like humans, seem much more reckless when they are young, and cats older than five years seem to possess enough common sense to keep them out of trouble. They realize that cars are dangerous, aggressive cats are to be avoided, and you shouldn't eat anything that you didn't catch yourself. Some people have allowed a very careful introduction into the pleasures of the outdoors by training their young cat to walk on a leash for trips around the yard or the park. Others find that their cat is willing to hang out close by while they garden or relax in the back yard. And some dedicated cat lovers have tried to provide the best of all worlds by creating expansive chicken-wire-and-lumber outdoor areas adjacent to their house where cats can sun-bathe, watch the bugs and birds, and smell the rich tapestry of life on the outside. Dr. Lappin, the famous cat doctor from CSU, has such an area where his cats can come and go as they please, warming the couches indoors when they choose and enjoying the smells of nature when the mood strikes. Lucky cats indeed.

One final, very important, caveat when it comes to providing the ideally enriched environment for your cat's well-being: Cats are all different. If you know and under-stand one cat...well, you understand one cat. Cats differ in personality and preferences, whether this is caused by the socialization from their mother and early kittenhood experiences, or whether their neurohormonal systems are simply geared differently. The most obvious divide is between the confident cats (referred to as "adrenaline junkies" in previous chapters) and the timid, shy cats (the "scaredy cats"). Enrichment means completely different things to these two personality types.

The confident cat craves more action. These are cats that thrive in the stimulating outdoor world, and when confined in the house they need a challenge, a chance to play, and the opportunity to explore different sights, sounds, and smells. The timid cat is likely to be stressed by spending time outdoors, and in the house this cat needs more hiding places, less sensory stimulation, and control over its interaction with other animals and people in the house. Both personalities need high perching areas; for the confident cat, this provides a throne from which it can survey its kingdom, while the timid cat uses it as a place to retreat safely above it all.

Every personality has its own needs and wants. We may not always be able to understand our cats, but sensitive observation may help us to adapt the environment to the needs of the individual cat.

Chapter 12: OLDER AND WISER

For a moment, Praline looked up casually toward the kitchen counter. Then with a slow but graceful leap the old cat jumped to the counter, her body a lithe symphony of short white and tabby fur covering a feline form whose bony contours were starting to show a little. She strolled across the counter and helped herself to a piece of bacon that was cooling by the stove. "Hey, what do you think you are doing?" Mike scolded. Praline knew the no-counter rule well, and in her younger years she would have never violated it (at least not when her owner was standing in plain view). But Praline was fifteen years old now, and she had cultivated an attitude of entitlement that many cats develop with age. She just looked at Mike and gave a little meow that seemed to say "Yeah, yeah, what are you going to do about it?" as she strolled to the end of the counter, jumped down, and carried the prize to her favorite corner of the room.

One of the charms of older cats is that they seem to become more human. Maybe this is because we have lived with the cat for so long that we intuitively understand them, as we might know a marriage partner of forty years. Or maybe it is because the cat understands us after a lifetime of observing our human ways. It may be that age has stripped away the drama and urgency of life, so that unimportant things can be ignored and the daily pleasures of life can be savored. Old age is the reward for having survived.

The "golden years" are much kinder to cats than they are to dogs, or even humans. The early years from two to five are the most stressful, as cats struggle to adapt to their environment, learn to cooperate with others (or not), and deal with "life on the edge". The middle years from five to ten years of age are usually uneventful, the prime of life and good health after having come to terms with their lifestyle. At ten years old things change as the finely tuned physiologic systems, designed for survival on the edge, start to slip a few notches. But the feline ability to invent and adapt gives the older cat a deep well of resources to draw upon as age creeps up. The stress-induced diseases tend to burn themselves out, or at least become more easily managed. Aging kidneys are less able to conserve water than they used to, but the cat increases its water consumption and starts to prefer more canned food to maintain its hydration. The cat that used to spend much of its time exploring the neighborhood shortens the outdoor visits to a little roaming and sniffing, strategically avoiding the times and places where other cats may challenge it. Life is good for an old cat.

Once a cat reaches ten years of age in good health it is reasonable to expect that it will live another full decade, but there will be health issues. This chapter is devoted to understanding the medical needs of cats and how they affect the length and quality of life. Some of these health problems are an expected part of feline aging, but the good thing about these common geriatric diseases is that they are mostly treatable, and in many cases curable. My favorite veterinary patient is the older cat. When a concerned owner presents their fourteen-year-old Siamese that has lost two pounds and vomits three times a week, I know that the cause of the problem will be easy to find with basic blood tests, and three months later the cat will have regained its weight and its attitude. The owner will be relieved to hear that they have another five years of their crotchety old cat waking them up each morning with its insistent meow. I can usually tell the owners "Yes, someday your cat will have a life-ending illness, but not this time." Nothing is better than seeing these same geriatric kitties well into their late teen years.

Before examining the things that we can do to make life better for the aging kitty, we need an introduction to the issues that nearly every cat will face in its second decade of life.

Diabetes mellitus, or "sugar diabetes", has become a common lifestyle-related disease of the overweight indoor cat. Feline diabetes is almost exclusively Type 2 Diabetes, the version in which excess body fat and stress block the ability of the body's insulin to control blood sugar. Cats are inherently susceptible to this condition, since they evolved for a low-carbohydrate diet that produces low and steady levels of blood sugar. But nearly every cat that weighs over fifteen pounds is likely to have prediabetic tendencies. Cat owners often insist that their beautiful eighteen pound male cat is "not overweight, he is just a big boy". And they may be right. But big cats are big because they produce large amounts of growth hormone, and growth hormone has its own insulin-blocking effects. Add a little extra body fat and a helping of stress hormones, and the healthy large cat can suddenly tip over into a diabetic crisis. The signs of diabetes may be vague at first; the increased thirst that is an early warning sign in humans and dogs is rarely noticed by cat owners, and most of the other aging diseases can also cause an increase in water drinking and urination. Sudden weight loss often occurs when the cat starts losing large amounts of sugar in its urine, but cat owners often take credit for getting their cat to lose extra pounds. "I switched him to a new brand of light food, and just look at him now," they say. But even a brief feel along the spine reveals that the cat has lost muscle and its skin has lost its sleek tautness. One of the common reasons that people bring their cat in for diagnosis is that their kitty has started urinating outside of the litter box. Most diabetics also have urinary infections, as bacteria thrive on the sugar passed in the urine, but there is a more interesting explanation for litter box avoidance proposed by Dr. Deborah Greco, of Colorado State University and the Animal Medical Center in New York City. Dr. Greco wondered if cats might develop the painful sensations that plague humans with diabetic neuropathy, in which nerve fibers in the hands and feet become simultaneously numb and painful. Imagine stepping into the litter box with prickly painful bare feet and it is easy to see why neuropathy would prompt any reasonable cat to pee somewhere more comfortable. When Dr. Greco biopsied the fine nerve fibers in the feet of diabetic cats she found that they looked just like the sensory nerves in humans with diabetic neuropathy. This raised the question of whether some cats that are not overtly diabetic might also have excessively sensitive feet, and it was subsequently discovered that some cats with blood sugar levels of 160-180 (most veterinarians would not diagnose diabetes unless the blood sugar was consistently above 220) already had nerve changes associated with diabetic neuropathy.

The treatment of diabetes in cats can be challenging. Although lifestyle and diet change can help many diabetic cats go into remission, insulin injections are required to overcome "glucose toxicity" and allow diet change and controlled weight loss to help. Prevention is the most effective strategy, and our prescription for every older large cat is simple: switch to a low-carbohydrate canned-food-only diet, encourage weight loss to less than fifteen pounds, avoid cortisone-containing medications (which can also trigger diabetes), and reduce the cat's stress level whenever possible. Fortunately, feline diabetes is the least common of four senior cat diseases.

The most interesting malady of older cats has environmental implications for humans. In the late 1970's veterinarians began to see older cats that were mysteriously losing weight and showing other vague symptoms that included a racing heart, nervousness, occasional vomiting, and increased water-drinking and urination. This disease looks like most of the other geriatric cat diseases, with a twist: the thyroid hormone levels in the blood are well above normal. Sometimes an enlarged thyroid gland can be felt in the jugular groove along the sides of the cat's neck, but since the normal thyroid glands are tucked in behind the trachea the lumps are not often noticeable. When these enlarged glands are biopsied, they are almost always benign thyroid tumors, which would not be dangerous except that they produce massive amounts of the hormone which controls metabolism. As a result, all of the cat's systems are stuck in high gear. No matter how much the cat eats, it will lose weight as the overactive metabolism burns up every available calorie, and then some.

The first case of hyperthyroidism that I diagnosed was my own cat. The year was 1978 and our beautiful long-haired Balinese cat appeared completely healthy at fifteen years of age. There was nothing about our kitty that concerned us, but when one of our other cats of the same age suddenly developed diabetes, we figured that a few blood tests on Blue Eyes would be reassuring. What we found was a thyroid hormone level four times the normal. One of her liver enzymes was also slightly elevated, and upon closer examination her heart rate was 240 beats per minute (anything heart rate over 200 attracts our attention, even in a nervous cat). Although she didn't appear too skinny, the scale showed that she had lost a little weight. Hyperthyroidism had just been reported in the veterinary journals, and armed with the description of this new disease, we knew what to do. Even then we had effective treatments that allowed Blue Eyes to recover her weight and her health.

Over the course of the past four decades hyperthyroidism has become progressively more common. Since Blue Eyes, almost every one of the fifteen cats that have shared our house has eventually developed hyperthyroidism. When researchers looked for a cause for this new disease, suspicion fell on something unknown in the environment, but the "smoking gun" was hard to pinpoint. The first clue was that cats eating mainly canned fish foods were ten times more likely to develop hyperthyroidism, as were those kitties fed from "pop-top" cans that didn't require a can opener[1]. The breakthrough came when investigators measured levels of chemicals called PolyBrominated-DiphenylEthers (PBDEs), which were used as flame retardants for carpeting, upholstery, and small electronic appliances starting in the 1970's. PBDEs were known to have hormone-disrupting effects, but previous studies had shown negligible levels of the chemicals in people's blood. But what about toddlers, who crawl all over the floor with their gooey little hands? And cats, that groom themselves constantly and swallow chemical-laden dust from the furniture and carpet? When these were measured the toddlers showed higher than adult levels of PBDEs in their blood, and some cats had twenty to one hundred times the normal human levels. Many of these cats developed hyperthyroidism, a highly suspicious link.

These chemicals have been on the list of environmental suspects for years, but proof is hard to come by, especially when the effects of a substance can take a decade to show effects. PBDEs are very stable, and they find their way into streams and oceans to build up concentrations in fish and other sea life. But even once the link between these chemicals and hormone problems is established, it isn't clear what can be done about cleaning up the environment. These chemicals have been outlawed in Europe for more than ten years and their use on carpeting and upholstery has declined in this country, but decontaminating our environment will be a gradual process. I always get a wry smile when I discuss this with female owners of hyperthyroid cats: "Tell your husband that you need to get all new furniture and carpet to eliminate these toxins in the house. It is for your cat's health!"

Perhaps in a decade or two these household chemicals will decrease enough that we will see less thyroid disease in older cats. In the meantime, hyperthyroid is the most common and treatable health problem of older cats. Medication can be used to decrease the production of hormone from the thyroid tumors, the hyperactive nodules can be removed with minor surgery, or the cat can receive a single injection of radioactive iodine, which internally radiates and kills only the abnormal cells. Iodine 131 treatment is the gold standard for treatment, but the cat must be kept in a nuclear medicine facility for up to a week until its urine is no longer radioactive. Each treatment has advantages and disadvantages, but even the fifteen-year-old kitty with heart problems, hypertension, and dramatic weight loss is likely to regain its health and live for another five years.

The weak link in the cat's marvelous system of organs is the kidneys, and any cat that lives well into its second decade will face age-related decline in kidney function. Since cats are built for life in the desert, it would seem like the kidneys should be the strongest organs in the body, conserving the body's water content and eliminating waste products with maximum efficiency. This is true for the younger cat, whose urine is concentrated to excrete minimal amounts of water and maximum amounts of nitrogen-containing waste. Cat urine is much more concentrated than that produced by humans or dogs. But high-performance systems can be more susceptible to wear and tear. Fortunately, all mammals are born with more functional kidney cells than needed. Over the course of our lives age takes its toll on the kidneys, but we can lose two-thirds of our urinary function with no discernible effect (which is why a person can donate one of their kidneys, which immediately decreases kidney function by half). As function drops below 30%, more water is lost in the urine and the urine becomes more dilute. For the cat owner, this means that they start to notice larger clumps of urine in the litter box and an increase in water consumption. At this point the kidneys can still do their primary job of excreting waste products, but once function drops below 25% then the body's toxins start to build up and affect the cat's health. Although the kidneys have forty other important functions (water regulation, electrolyte balance, production of hormones to regulate blood pressure, stimulation of red blood cell production, and conservation of protein and other nutrients), the blood tests that measure waste product levels reflect only the most obvious functions of the urinary system. Kidney deterioration is a gradual process that becomes evident only in old age, and we have traditionally accepted this as an inevitable cost of increasing years. This approach of "we have to expect that the kidneys will fail with age" is probably not fair to our geriatric feline friends, and we are starting to understand that the progression of renal failure may not be inevitable. There are some predictable changes as kidney function decreases, and many of the these can be controlled.

The extremely concentrated urine of the normal cat prevents infection, but as the urine becomes more dilute with age bacteria can move up the urinary tract and establish chronic low-grade infection ("pyelonephritis") in the urine-collecting areas of the kidneys. Many cats over ten years old have hidden urinary infection. Even though these cats do not appear sick, controlling kidney infection will delay further kidney deterioration.

As more water is passed by the aging kidneys, more potassium is lost in the urine. Low potassium levels are very common in older cats and the symptoms are vague, but we now understand that decreased potassium further impairs kidney function. Low potassium also causes muscular weakness and pain, and many creaky old cats that act like they are arthritic actually have hypokalemia, a decrease in potassium in the cells. Fortunately, extra potassium can be supplemented with the food to replace the loss of this electrolyte, and the results of this simple addition can dramatically improve the cat's well-being.

High blood pressure is another complication of age and declining kidney function, a hidden killer that has not received enough attention in older cats. Blood pressure measurement is tricky in dogs and cats and getting an accurate reading is more difficult in smaller animals. Cats don't enjoy their veterinary visits, so the "white coat effect" of anxiety in the veterinary office further complicates the situation. In severe cases, high blood pressure can cause detachment of the retina and sudden blindness, but in most cases the effects of increased BP are gradual deterioration in the brain and kidneys. Once high blood pressure is identified, it can usually be controlled.

As the aging kidneys lose more water and electrolytes in the urine, it becomes more difficult for the cat to stay hydrated. A simple test for dehydration is to lift a fold of loose skin over the shoulder area and release it; if the cat is well-hydrated the skin will return to its normal position within two seconds. If the skin stays tented up, the cat is at least 5% dehydrated. Dehydration can occur even when the cat is drinking copious amounts of water. Dehydration is not really about water, but rather about the electrolytes that control fluid balance in the body. In some cats with serious dehydration issues, owners can learn to give subcutaneous injections of an electrolyte solution (your vet can provide the fluids, tubing, and needles) once or twice a week to maintain fluid balance and normal blood pH, and this simple treatment can have dramatic effects on older cats whose health is failing.

Finally, diet plays an important part in kidney function, which brings up another controversy. It has long been recognized that the most important waste products that the kidney eliminates are the breakdown products of dietary protein. At one time there was a popular theory that too much dietary protein would "wear out" the kidneys, but this has been disproven. It does seem to be true that in advanced kidney failure the level of toxic wastes can be lowered by a feeding low protein diet, and prescription "kidney diets" are designed with this in mind. As veterinarians we have been guilty of the mistake of prescribing low protein diets for old cats in the early stages of kidney disease; more recent work suggests that cats with moderately compromised kidneys actually do better on a high protein diet until they reach an advanced stage of renal failure. Some nutritionists feel that the positive effects of prescription kidney diets are not due to low protein, but to low phosphorus (regulation of phosphorus and calcium is impaired in kidney disease, and phosphorus is toxic to the kidneys) and the generous supplementation of B vitamins that these diets include.

Although the physiology of aging kidneys is complicated, we can use our new understanding to make adjustments and slow the progression of the disease and improve the quality of life for the senior cat:

1. Control kidney infection; often periodic "pulse therapy" of antibiotics is preferable to waiting for infection to become obvious and repeatedly culturing the urine.
2. Supplement potassium if blood tests show even borderline low levels.
3. Control high blood pressure.
4. Prevent and treat dehydration with fresh water, canned food (which contains 80% moisture), and subcutaneous fluid treatment if needed.
5. Choose a quality diet that has extra potassium and lower levels of phosphorus; many "senior cat diets" are appropriate.

The endearing charms of older cats make the necessary medical tinkering well worthwhile. The sense of entitlement that older cats develop is well-deserved. Younger cats may be demanding, but older cats know that they are worth it, and have become expert in manipulating others to get what they deserve. Perhaps "manipulate" is too negative a term. Often these behaviors have been carefully negotiated in relationships with the humans and other cats in the household.

Rituals are particularly valued by the older cat, and it can be helpful to consciously create routines that increase the cat's sense of predictability. It is reassuring to have expectations that are understood and met. Food is always a bridge in any relationship, and many owners will reserve some small treat for a daily feline event. One cat person I know pours herself a glass of wine at 8 o'clock each evening, just as she sits down to watch a little prime-time television. She taps the edge of her wine glass as a distinctive sound signal, and when her kitty jumps on her lap, she gives him one small cocktail shrimp, followed by a short petting session. As one might expect, her cat seems to know and anticipate this little daily dose of pleasure, and at 7:59 he can be found restlessly meowing around his owner's favorite chair to remind her of their date. Other cats have their own routines: drinking out of the sink at bedtime, or five minutes of play with a "kitty tease" when the person arrives home from work.

Routines and rituals are particularly useful as the feline brain ages. As many cats approach twenty years of age, signs of senility start to appear and routine is welcome as the mind starts to lose its fine edge. It isn't always easy to tell if your eighteen-year-old kitty is losing its marbles. House-training lapses may be caused by confusion, but there may also be physical reasons, such as being too stiff to get in and out of the litter box. Wandering the house restlessly during the evening hours may be a type of confusion similar to the "Sundowner Syndrome" shown by human Alzheimer's patients, but it may just be that the demanding old cat is just hoping for another feeding, or patrolling it's indoor territory more because it smelled a new cat out in the neighborhood. Unlike senile dogs that are often are plagued by anxiety as they develop cognitive dysfunction, senile cats seem to be undisturbed by the loss of brain function, remaining happily enveloped in a Zen-like state of acceptance.

One of the most distinctive behaviors of feline senility is aimless nocturnal vocalization. At least once a week my old cat Snowy would jolt me out of deep sleep around midnight with a piercing yowl. From his volume and tone I immediately thought that a bookcase had fallen on him or he was suffering the intense pain of a blood clot blocking the artery to his rear legs (imagining the worst is a hazard of knowing too much about medicine). I would leap out of bed, my own heart pounding, and race out to the living room, only to find Snowy standing in the middle of the room as if in a trance. I would reach down to stroke his head to see if he was OK, and he would simply look up at me with a look of recognition that seemed to say "Oh, you're up! How nice". After a few pets he would purr and wander off, and I would return to bed with my heart still racing, to try to recapture sleep.

Not every cat that yowls in the night for no reason is confused and senile. When technologic advances made it easier to measure blood pressure in cats, we discovered that some cats with nocturnal vocalization also had hypertension, and when the blood pressure was controlled the nightly vocal outbursts ceased. This connection is easy to overlook, even for veterinarians. Jazzmine was our Siamese cross, with tortoiseshell points and pale blue eyes. We had adopted her as a kitten, and she lived with us for eighteen years. Her only health problem was Lymphocytic Stomatitis, a painful mouth problem in which the immune system creates intense inflammation of the gums and ultimately eats away the enamel of the teeth. Over the years we removed one tooth after another as these cavity-like lesions surrounded by red, swollen gums ravaged her mouth. Once all of her teeth had been removed the condition was gone, but the stress of chronic pain had left her with some sort of mental illness. She became a recluse, blocking out everything around her with an invisible wall. Jazzmine would adopt a small spot, such as under the fireplace hearth, where she could be found at all times. She seemed content when she narrowed her world down to a few square feet. Although her chosen spot was in plain view, she seemed to think that nobody could see her. If we reached into her spot to touch her she was clearly startled, as if her invisibility cloak was pulled away, and she would leave her "safe spot" for someplace new. Eventually we learned to go along with her "hiding in plain sight", and even the other cats in our house ignored her; perhaps they had some sense that she was a few kibbles short of a full bowl. In her fifteenth year, Jazzmine started having episodes of yowling at night. Although the link between nocturnal vocalization and hypertension had been well described and I had diagnosed many cases of hypertensive yowling in my patients, I assumed that Jazzmine was simply developing dementia to go with her other mental issues and I didn't check her blood pressure. Eventually one of my associate veterinarians chided me: "You always tell people to have their cat's blood pressure checked when they do this. Haven't you measured Jazzmine's?" Sometimes things are more obvious to someone who hasn't lived with your old cat every day for years. When we finally measured her blood pressure, it turned out that her BP was well over 200; once we started her on blood pressure medicine the pressure dropped to 150 and the yowling stopped. She remained a strange cat for the rest of her years, but happy enough if we respected her few square feet of secret territory.

We met Praline at the beginning of this chapter, and she taught me about another reason for cats that sing in the night. When she was seventeen years old, her owners asked me about her habit of vocalizing in a quavery Katharine Hepburn-like voice after the lights were out and everyone had gone to bed. Praline was a quirky old kitty, but her health checked out fine: No sign of early diabetes, no pain that we could find, and blood pressure comfortably within the normal range. As we discussed the episodes further, her owners mentioned that Praline was always in the same place when she yowled at the top of her voice. They lived in a large house, and the rounded foyer was a full two stories high, the acoustically perfect spot to amplify her voice. Apparently Praline intentionally sought this perfect venue for her singing. Perhaps her hearing was diminished and she wanted the reassurance of hearing herself, or maybe this was just another idiosyncratic pleasure, like a person belting out ABBA songs in the shower.

Cats of all ages can have strong opinions about their food, and the finicky feline is almost a cliché. Food preferences take on a new twist in some older cats and owners of senior kitties often complain that their cat, which has happily eaten the same food for years, is now refusing its regular diet. When offered a new flavor of food it will gobble it eagerly, but after a period of time it will turn away and refuse the food. "Maybe she gets tired of the same food?" the owner asks, but there is more to it. A phenomenon called "acquired food aversion" occurs in many animals (including humans), but it is particularly common in old cats. Many of us can relate: when we experience an evening of stomach flu we may lose our appetite for whatever food we had for dinner, even though the food was not responsible. Food aversion is a useful protective mechanism; if the brain can make a connection between nausea and the most recent thing that was ingested then it keeps the animal from making the mistake again. Sometimes the connection is temporal and not cause-and-effect, but the brain figures it is better to be safe than sorry.

Many of the health issues that affect older cats can cause nausea, even if no vomiting occurs. Mild kidney disease, inflammatory bowel disease, chronic pancreatitis, and other vague "don't feel so good" illnesses can give the cat that feeling of "it must have been something I ate", creating an aversion to the most recent flavor of food that was eaten. The feeling of stomach upset passes quickly, but the cat will continue to refuse that food, even when it is hungry. Once we recognize this phenomenon, we can deal with it by offering food that tastes different from the food that was refused. Unfortunately, the same thing may happen to the new food if nausea returns, so cat owners need to develop a sense of when to change food and when to stick with the familiar diet. One practical application of this principle comes when a seriously ill cat is recovering from an illness. The conscientious veterinarian may prescribe a special diet to keep intestinal disease from flaring up again or to help control kidney waste products, but we sometimes make the mistake of introducing the new food before the stomach upset is completely resolved. If we give a food that may be beneficial in the long run before the cat's nausea resolves, we simply guarantee that the cat will find it disgusting. Once again, improving the cat's quality of life depends on giving the cat what it wants—even if the cat itself doesn't know what that is.

Despite the challenges of chronic health problems, older cats are often living the best years of their lives. They have come to terms with life, feeling secure in their home and their relationships with their people and other cat and dog friends that share their lives.

Mike always had stories to tell me about Praline as she aged gracefully. She developed a love for watching college basketball on TV (the squeak of sneakers on hardwood seemed to remind the remote corners of her predatory brain of mousy voices), and she continue to sing in the foyer every night. She became skilled at manipulating the younger cats with either an intense stare or a pretension of complete indifference. Praline didn't groom herself as well as she had when she was younger, but she loved to have her owners brush her thoroughly every evening. When Mike switched her to canned food, she loved the sensory banquet of smells, tastes, and textures, and looked forward to every meal. Every afternoon nap became a pleasure and every affectionate petting became another reason to enjoy the good life.

EPILOGUE

What is it like to be a cat? We can never really know. All members of the cat family have evolved to fit a demanding, no-room-for-compromise lifestyle that is foreign to us. While dogs and humans have the luxury of organizing group activities, chewing on toys for hours, or pondering the meaning of life, cats are designed to attack life and live it. While this gives cats the reputation of being independent, self-centered, and even selfish, the fact that cats can step out of their life-on-the-edge world to show affection, learn new behaviors, and thrive in a human environment should inspire us to stretch our own limits.

The internet is littered with posts about "What We Can Learn From Our Cats". Apparently bloggers have nothing better to do than stare at their cat, hoping for material for their next column. Most of the dozens of lessons that we are supposed to learn from our cat are shallow clichés based on how we might feel if we could lay around all day with nothing to do: "It is always time for another nap", "Know who loves you and who feeds you", "Teach people how to treat you", "Don't always do what people want you to do", "Live in the moment", "Sunshine is the best therapy" (well, maybe we should listen to this last one). What our fascination with lessons from our cats does reveal is their "otherness"; cats are not the same as us, and they prompt us to question whether we could do things differently, especially when change upsets our world.

One of my favorite cartoons appeared in a magazine many years ago. It showed a variation on an old caricature of human evolution. At the left is a primordial fish climbing out of the ocean on its fins. The thought balloon above its head reads "Eat. Survive. Reproduce." To its right are two more developed creatures with legs and tails. Their thought balloons read "Eat. Survive. Reproduce." In the center of the frame is a hairy ape-like creature stooped over and walking on its knuckles. The thought balloon above its head reads "Eat. Survive. Reproduce." Finally at the right side of the cartoon is a modern human in slacks and a sweater-vest. As he gazes off into the distance, the thought balloon above his head reads "What is it all about?" Perhaps the lesson we can learn from our cats is to take one step back from the right side of the cartoon and understand that the meaning of life may be simply to live life.

The focus of this book has to improve the quality of our cats' lives by understanding their needs and providing an environment in which they can thrive. In order to do this, we need to appreciate that even the most placid cat may be a seething cauldron of emotion and stress hormones any time there is change in the house, conflict with other animals, or too much sensory stimulation. There is no boundary between physical and mental health, and the cat's emotions are reflected in physical changes throughout its body. The quality of a cat's life is a finely balanced mixture of brain and body, food and friends, senses and recreation. Cats are famous for their independence, but they rely upon us to provide this balance.

At the beginning of this book I introduced my cat Ania, perched comfortably on the back of our couch, gazing out the window at the new-fallen snow in our yard. I don't know what was going through her mind. Was she soothed by the quiet peacefulness of the snow-covered neighborhood, or did the sudden unfamiliarity of the sight make her feel like her world was ending? Ania had been prone to health problems, including a short period of stress-induced heart failure and recurring pancreatitis attacks, so I wondered if she might develop some illness in the next few days. But those physical problems are all behind her, and as she nears her twentieth year she is healthy and I truly believe that she is living the Good Life. When I walk into the living room on this particular morning, Ania turns her head to look at me, gives a long stretch, and ambles over to ask for a little scratch on a favorite spot under her chin. Then she settles into a small patch of sunshine coming through the window.

ACKNOWLEDGEMENTS

A debt of gratitude is owed to all of the cats I have known and all of the cat lovers who have shared their stories with me over the past four decades. I have learned from all of them.

Veterinarians, naturalists, behaviorists, and researchers have offered invaluable insights into cat health and behavior and their contributions are appreciated.

Many people have helped in this project. Don Culver sifted through each word for clarity and punctuation. Jamie Bozzi, a behavioral consultant with smrtdog.com, has offered her comments and Dr. Yvette Virgin with Sacajawea Healthcare for Pets has given the manuscript a critical reading. Peggy Sue Kittrick used her expertise to proof and format the final draft. Linda Legg contributed the cover photo of her cat J.W. Tuffer Harris and Landon Gordon assisted in the photography, design, and graphics of the cover.

Finally, this project could not have been completed without the constant support and encouragement of my wife, Terri Culver. Thank you.

THE GOOD LIFE FOR CATS: References

The books and articles listed are selected from the thousands of references that attempt to explain cats, the brain, and the complexities of medicine. When statistics are quoted, it can be helpful to show where they were published, and when new concepts and observations are presented readers may want to learn more from those sources.

GENERAL READING REFERENCES

[A]"The Tribe of Tiger: Cats And Their Culture", by Elizabeth Marshall Thomas, Simon and Schuster, copyright 1994 by Jared Taylor Williams

[B] "Making Rounds with Oscar: The Extraordinary Gift of An Ordinary Cat", by Dr. David Dosa, Hyperion ebooks, copyright 2010 by David Dosa

[C]"The Cat's Mind: Understanding Your Cat's Behavior", by Bruce Fogle, DVM, MRCVS, Macmillan, copyright 1992 by Bruce Fogle

[D]"Cat Culture: The Social World Of A Cat Shelter", by Janet M. Alger and Steven F. Alger, Temple University Press, copyright 2003 by Temple University

[E] "The Polyvagal Theory: Neurophysiological Foundations of Emotions, Attachment, Communication, Self-Regulation", by Stephen W. Porges, W W Norton and Company, Copyright 2011 by Stephen W. Porges

[F] "The Cat Who Cried For Help", by Nicholas Dodman, DVM, Bantam Books, copyright 1997 by Nicholas Dodman

[G] "Balance: In Search of the Lost Sense", by Scott McCredie, Little, Brown and Company, copyright 2007 by Scott McCredie

PREFACE

[1] E. Roy John, Phyllis Chesler, Frank Barlett, Ira Victor, Observation Learning in Cats, Science, March 29, 1968, vol 159, Issue 3822, pp1489-1491

CHAPTER 1: Life on the Edge

[1] Charlotte O Ladd, Revecca L Huot, KV Thrivikraman, Charles B Nemeroff, Michael J Meany, and Pual M. Plotsky, Long-term behavioral and neuroendocrine adaptations to adverse early experience, Progress in Brain Research, Vol 122, Ch 7, Elsevier Science

[2] Paul M. Plotsky, Postnatal experience alters hypothalamic corticotropin-releasing factor (CRF) mRNA, median eminence CRF content, and stress-induced release in rats, Molecular Brain Research, Vol 18, Issue 3, May 1993, pp195-200

[3] Mila Roceri, Francesca Cirulli, Cassandra Pessina, Paolo Peretto, Giorgio Rasagni, Marco A Riva, Postnatal repeated

maternal deprivation produces age-dependent changes of brain-derived neurotrophic factor expression in selected rat brain regions, Biological Psychiatry, April 2004, Vol 55, Issue 7, pp708-714

[4] Robert M Sapolsky, Mothering style and methylation, Nature Neuroscience 7, 2004, pp791-792

[5] Maria L Boccia, Cort A Pedersen, Brief vs long maternal separations in infancy: contrasting relationships with adult maternal behavior and lactating levels of aggression and anxiety, Psychoneuroendocrinology, Vol 26, Issue 7, Oct 2001, pp657-672

CHAPTER 2: Ways of Knowing

[1] Lori R. Kogan, Regina Schoenfeld-Tacher, and Peter W Hellyer, Cats in Animal Shelters: Exploring the Common Perception that Black Cats Take Longer to Adopt, The Open Veterinary Science Journal, 2013, 7, 18-22

[2] Thomas Nagel, What is it like to be a bat?, From The Philosophical Review LXXXIII, 4 October 1974, pp435-50

[3] MT Wallace, MA Meredith, and BE Stein, Converging influences from visual, auditory, and somatosensory cortices onto output neurons of the superior colliculus, Journal of Neurophysiology, June 1, 1993 Vol. 69 no. 6, pp1797-1809

[4] Cerissa A. Griffith, BS; Elizabeth S. Steigerwald, PhD; C. A. Tony Buffington, DVM, PhD, DACVN, Effects of a synthetic facial pheromone Journal of the American Veterinary Medical Association, October 15, 2000, Vol. 217, No. 8, Pages 1154-1156

[5]Weiwei Lei, Aurore Ravoninjohary, Xia Li, Robert F. Margolskee, Danielle R. Reed, Gary K. Beauchamp,Peihua Jiang. Functional Analyses of Bitter Taste Receptors in Domestic Cats (Felis catus). PLOS ONE, 2015; 10 (10): e0139670

CHAPTER 3: Secret Senses

[1]Davide Castelvecchi, The Compass Within, Scientific American, January 2012 306, pp48-53

CHAPTER 5: A Sense of Place

[1]P Bernstein, M Strack, Home Ranges, Favored Spots, Time-sharing Patterns, and Tail Usage by 14 Cats in the Home, Animal Behavior Consultants Newsletter, 1993

CHAPTER 6: What's for Dinner?

[1]PD Pion, MD Kittleson, QR Rogers, JG Morris Myocardial failure in cats associated with low plasma taurine: a reversible cardiomyopathy, Science 14 Aug 1987: Vol. 237, Issue 4816, pp. 764-768

[2]Nicole Bennett, DVM, MS, ACVIM , Deborah S. Greco, DVM, PhD, et al, Comparison of a low carbohydrate–low fiber diet and a moderate carbohydrate–high fiber diet in the management of
feline diabetes mellitus, Journal of Feline Medicine & Surgery Volume 8, Issue 2, April 2006, Pages 73–84

[3] Claudia Wallis, Gut Reactions, Scientific American, June 2014, pp30-33

CHAPTER 7: New Ways and Old Ways

[1] David C. Grant, DVM, Effect of water source on intake and urine
concentration in healthy cats, Journal of Feline Medicine and Surgery, June 2010 vol. 12 no. 6 431-434

[2] Seefeldt SL , Chapman TE Body water content and turnover in cats fed dry and canned rations. American Journal of Veterinary Research, 1979, 40(2):183-185

CHAPTER 8: The Inside Story

[1] John Bienenstock et al at McMaster University, Hamilton, Canada, and John Cryan at University College Cork, Ireland, as reported in Science News, October 8, 2011, p9 (probiotics, stress, and vagus)

[2] Norsworthy GD, Estep JS, KiupelM, et al. Diagnosis of chronic small bowel disease in cats: 100 cases (2008-2012). Journal of American Veterinary Medical Association 2013;243<10):1455-1461.

[3] Elizabeth R. Bertone, Laura A. Snyder, and Anthony S. Moore, Environmental Tobacco Smoke and Risk of Malignant Lymphoma in Pet Cats American Journal of Epidemiology, August 1, 2002, 156: 268-73

[4] SN Bybee, AV Scorza, MR Lappin, Effect of the probiotic SF68 on presence of diarrhea in cats and dogs housed in an animal shelter, Journal of the American College of Internal Medicine, 2011; 25:pp856-860

CHAPTER 9: Let's Be Friends—Or Not!

[1] The Cambridge Declaration on Consciousness, written by Philip Lowe, edited by Jaak Panksepp, Diana Reiss, David

Edelman, Bruno Van Swinderen, Philip Low, and Christof Koch, announced by Stephen Hawking, July 7, 2012. Available at www.fcmconference.org/img/CambridgeDeclarationOnConsciousness.pdf

[2]Dawn E. Frazer Sissom, D. A. Rice , G. Peters, How Cats Purr, Journal of Zoology, January 1991

[3]Karen McComb, , Anna M. Taylor, Christian Wilson, Benjamin D. Charlton, The Cry Embedded Within the Purr, Current Biology, Volume 19, Issue 13, 14 July 2009, Pages R507–R508

[4]Anthony Lewis Wigram, The Effects of Vibroacoustic Therapy on Clinical and Non-Clinical Populations, Thesis submitted for degree of Doctor of Philosophy, St Georges Hospital Medical School

CHAPTER 10: Pandora's Problem

[1]Judi Stella, Candace Croneya, Tony Buffington, Effects of stressors on the behavior and physiology of domestic cats, Applied Animal Behaviour ScienceVolume 143, Issues 2–4, 31 January 2013, Pages 157–163
[2]C A T Buffington, Idiopathic Cystitis in Domestic Cats—Beyond the Lower
Urinary Tract, Journal of Veterinary Internal Medicine, 2011;25:784-196

[3]C A Tony Buffington,Jodi L Westropp, Dennis J Chew, From FUS to Pandora syndrome
Where are we, how did we get here, and where to now?,Journal of Feline Medicine and Surgery May 2014 vol. 16 no. 5 385-394

[4]C.A. Tony Buffington, Bunyen Teng, George T. Somogyi, Norepinephrine Content And Adrenoceptor Function In The Bladder Of Cats With Feline Interstitial Cystitis, The Journal of Urology, Volume 167, Issue 4, April 2002, Pages 1876–1880

[5]C.A. T. Buffington, Karel Pacak, Increased Plasma Norepinephrine Concentration In Cats With Interstitial Cystitis, The Journal of Urology, Volume 165, Issue 6, Part 1, June 2001, Pages 2051–2054

[6]Buffington, C A T, Developmental Influences on Medically Unexplained
Symptoms, Psychotherapeutics and Psychosomatics, Vol. 78, No. 3, April 2009, 78:139–144

CHAPTER 11: To The Good Life

[1]Sarah L H Ellis, Ilona Rodan, Hazel C Carney,Sarah Heath, Irene Rochlitz, Lorinda D Shearburn, Eliza Sundahl, Jodi L Westropp, AAFP and ISFM, Feline Environmental Needs Guidelines, Journal of Feline Medicine and Surgery, March 2013 vol. 15 no. 3 219-230

[2]Meghan E. Herron, DVM, DACVB and C. A. Tony Buffington, DVM, PhD, DACVN, Environmental Enrichment for Indoor Cats: Implementing Enrichment
Compendium of Continuing Education for Veterinarians. 2012 Jan; 34(1): E3.

[3]Horn, J. A., Mateus-Pinilla, N., Warner, R. E. and Heske, E. J. (2011), Home range, habitat use, and activity patterns of free-roaming domestic cats. The Journal of Wildlife Management, 75: 1177–1185.

[4]Jacqueline Neilsen, DVM, The Latest Scoop on Litter, Veterinary Practice, March 2009, pp140-144

CHAPTER 12: Older And Wiser

[1]Charlotte H. Edinboro, DVM, PhD J. Catharine Scott-Moncrieff, VetMB, MS, DACVIM, et al, Epidemiologic study of relationships between consumption of commercial canned food and risk of hyperthyroidism in cats, Journal of the American Veterinary Medical Association, March 15, 2004, Vol. 224, No. 6, Pages 879-886

[2]Janice A. Dye, Marta Venier, Lingyan Zhu, et al, Elevated PBDE Levels in Pet Cats: Sentinels for Humans?Environmental Science and Technology, 2007, 41 (18), pp 6350–6356

[3]Elizabeth R. Bertone, Laura A. Snyder, and Antony S. Moore, Environmental Tobacco Smoke and Risk of Malignant Lymphoma in Pet Cats, American Journal of Epidemiology,
(2002) 156 (3): 268-273

ABOUT THE AUTHOR

Dr. Lee R. Harris graduated from the Washington State University College of Veterinary Medicine in 1974 and has spent more than four decades caring for pets in his own multi-doctor veterinary hospital near Seattle and at other clinics in San Diego, Phoenix, and Seattle. A lifelong interest in animal behavior, neuroscience, human medicine, and psychology has given him a broad view of subjects relevant to the understanding of the feline patients that he loves. Dr. Harris has spoken and written extensively about cats and dogs, including articles in the Washington Post, Time Magazine, and the Houston Chronicle, as well as his book on canine lifestyle, "The Good Life for Dogs: health, lifestyle, happiness and meaning".

www.ingramcontent.com/pod-product-compliance
Lightning Source LLC
Chambersburg PA
CBHW060841280326
41934CB00007B/875